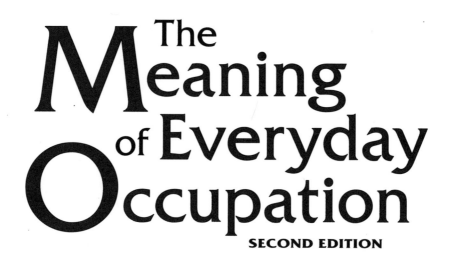

# The Meaning of Everyday Occupation

SECOND EDITION

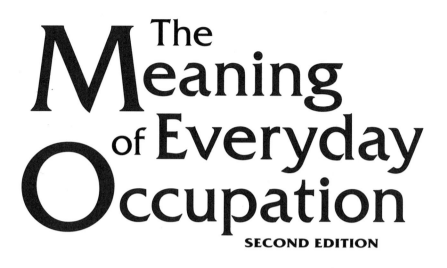

# The Meaning of Everyday Occupation

**SECOND EDITION**

Betty Risteen Hasselkus, PhD, OTR, FAOTA

Emeritus Professor
University of Wisconsin
Madison, Wisconsin

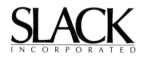

**SLACK**
INCORPORATED

www.slackbooks.com

ISBN: 978-1-55642-934-7
Copyright © 2011 by Betty Risteen Hasselkus

Cover and Chapter 1 photograph, Longenecker Gardens, University of Wisconsin Arboretum. © Zane Williams, Madison, WI.

Chapters 2, 4, 5, 6 photographs used with permission of Jim Sykes, Madison, WI.

Chapter 3 photograph used with permission of John Hasselkus.

Chapter 7 photograph used with permission of DO-IT Center, University of Washington.

Chapter 8, 9, 10 photographs used with permission of Richard Edic, Rochester, NY.

*The Meaning of Everyday Occupation, Second Edition Instructor's Manual* is also available from SLACK Incorporated. Don't miss this important companion to *The Meaning of Everyday Occupation, Second Edition* available at http://www.efacultylounge.com.

SLACK Incorporated uses a review process to evaluate submitted material. Prior to publication, educators or clinicians provide important feedback on the content that we publish. We welcome feedback on this work.

Library of Congress Cataloging-in-Publication Data

Hasselkus, Betty Risteen, 1939-
  The meaning of everyday occupation / Betty Risteen Hasselkus. -- 2nd ed.
    p. ; cm.
  Includes bibliographical references and index.
  ISBN 978-1-55642-934-7
  1. Occupational therapy--Philosophy.  I. Title.
  [DNLM: 1. Occupational Therapy--psychology. 2. Adaptation, Psychological. 3. Culture. 4. Interpersonal Relations. 5. Professional-Patient Relations. 6. Social Values. WB 555]
  RM735.H34 2011
  615.8'515--dc22
                                    2010043448

Published by:       SLACK Incorporated
                    6900 Grove Road
                    Thorofare, NJ 08086 USA
                    Telephone: 856-848-1000
                    Fax: 856-848-6091
                    www.slackbooks.com

Contact SLACK Incorporated for more information about other books in this field or about the availability of our books from distributors outside the United States.

Last digit is print number: 10  9  8  7  6  5  4  3  2  1

# CONTENTS

*About the Author* ............................................................................. *vii*
*Acknowledgments* ............................................................................. *ix*
*Introduction* ..................................................................................... *xi*

**Chapter 1    Meaning: An Essential for Life** ................................................. 1
    Personal and Social Meanings ............................................... 4
    Meaning and Performance in Life .......................................... 6
    Aspects of Seeing .................................................................. 8
    How Do We "Know" Meaning? ............................................ 10
    The Open Door Policy .......................................................... 14

**Chapter 2    Meaning in Everyday Occupation** ........................................... 19
    Happiness Is ... ..................................................................... 21
    Occupation and Being .......................................................... 25
    Occupation and Becoming .................................................... 29
    Occupation and Belonging .................................................... 32

**Chapter 3    Space and Place: Sources of Meaning in Occupation** ............ 39
    Space and Place in Our Lives ............................................... 41
    Health and Well-Being Within Space and Place .................... 42
    Space and Therapy ............................................................... 43
    From Space to Place in Therapy ........................................... 44
    Placelessness ........................................................................ 45
    A Place to Call Home ........................................................... 46
    Special Places ....................................................................... 51
    A Geography of Health ......................................................... 55

**Chapter 4    Culture and Occupation: The Experience of Similarity
                    and Difference** ........................................................................ 61
    Culture as Similarity and Difference ..................................... 63
    Cultivating the Similar in Our Lives ..................................... 67
    Cultivating Difference in Our Lives ...................................... 70
    Structuring the Similarities: Routines, Habits, and Rituals .... 71
    Disability as Difference ........................................................ 76

**Chapter 5    Occupation as a Source of Well-Being and Development** ...... 83
    The Essence of Well-Being ................................................... 85
    Occupation and Human Development .................................... 91
    Occupation to the End .......................................................... 96

**Chapter 6    Occupation as Meaningful Connection** ................................ 101
    Relation and the Professional ............................................. 103
    Relation and Well-Being ..................................................... 106
    Occupational Forms of Relation ......................................... 109
    Occupational Therapy and Connectedness .......................... 113

**Chapter 7    Disability and Occupation**................................................**123**
    The Faces of Disability.........................................126
    Occupation as Disability Experience .................................129
    Disability as Occupational Experience...............................133
    Being the Bridge ..........................................136

**Chapter 8    Occupation as a Source of Spirituality** ...............................**143**
    This Thing Called Spirituality.................................145
    Spiritual "Health"..........................................146
    Spirituality and Occupation: Compatible Partners? ...........................148
    Spirituality and Everyday Occupation .....................................150
    Spirituality and Occupational Therapy ...............................154
    The Space Within..........................................157

**Chapter 9    Creativity in Occupation as a Source of Meaning** ...........................**163**
    Creativity From Without and Within.................................166
    Arising From Chaos..........................................170
    Creativity and Health .......................................172
    To the Dancing Star .......................................179

**Chapter 10 Occupation Speaks: Final Thoughts** ...............................**183**
    The Therapist and the Splint...............................186

*Index* ........................................................*189*

# ABOUT THE AUTHOR

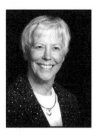 *Betty Risteen Hasselkus, PhD, OTR, FAOTA* is an Emeritus Professor of Kinesiology/Occupational Therapy at the University of Wisconsin–Madison where she served as program director for 10 years. Prior to her faculty appointment, she earned a bachelor of science degree in occupational therapy, a master of science degree in physical education, and a doctor of philosophy degree at the University of Wisconsin. The hospital where she did much of her training and where she held her first position in occupational therapy is also the building where she was born, where her children were born, and where, ultimately, the academic program of occupational therapy was located during her faculty years.

During her more than 40 years of active participation in the profession of occupational therapy, Dr. Hasselkus has focused her research, teaching, and practice on the everyday occupational experience of people in the community, with a special emphasis on family caregiving for older family members, physician–family caregiver relationships, meanings of everyday occupation to dementia daycare staff, and the meaning of doing occupational therapy. She was elected to the American Occupational Therapy Association Roster of Fellows in 1986 and to the American Occupational Therapy Foundation Academy of Research in 1999. Dr. Hasselkus was the invited Wilma West Lecturer at the University of Southern California in 2003, presenting a lecture entitled, "The Voice of Everyday Occupation." In 2005, she was awarded the AOTA Eleanor Clarke Slagle Lectureship Award—the Association's highest award for scholarship—and subsequently gave the award lecture in 2006, "The World of Everyday Occupation: Real People, Real Lives."

Dr. Hasselkus was editor of *The American Journal of Occupational Therapy* from 1998 to 2003. Her international reputation as a scholar has taken her to Australia, Canada, Sweden, Denmark, Wales, and Northern Ireland, where she has provided lectures and workshops on qualitative research methods, critical analysis, writing, and qualitative research opportunities in everyday occupation. Her scholarly career includes more than 90 publications in journals and texts.

# ACKNOWLEDGMENTS

My thanks go out to a number of people who have contributed in a variety of ways to this revised second edition of *The Meaning of Everyday Occupation*—special friends and colleagues Virginia Dickie and Elizabeth Crepeau, Karen Hammell with whom I feel a strong kindred spirit, photographer Richard Edic, John Hasselkus for his computer savvy, Landon Risteen for his editorial prowess, and granddaughter Julia for good-naturedly spending an entire morning on the swing in order to get a good photo for Chapter 3.

# INTRODUCTION

If you have taken this rubble for my past
raking through it for fragments you could sell
know that I long ago moved on
deeper into the heart of the matter

If you think you can grasp me, think again:
my story flows in more than one direction
a delta springing from the riverbed
with its five fingers spread

"Delta," *from TIME'S POWER: Poems 1985-1988 by Adrienne Rich.
Copyright © 1989 by Adrienne Rich. Used by permission of the author and
W.W. Norton & Company, Inc.*

This is a book about meaning and everyday occupation. Although such a topic may seem rather simple and straightforward, and *meaning* and *everyday occupation* may seem like self-evident concepts, upon closer inspection, it quickly becomes apparent that meaning and everyday occupation are many-faceted phenomena that deserve thoughtful and contextual discussion. They represent dimensions of being that are of the utmost importance to quality of life for each one of us. For if we do not have ordinary and familiar occupations in our daily lives, and if these occupations do not have personal significance to us, then, who *are* we and what is the purpose of life? How could any semblance of quality of life manifest itself in a world of nothingness and insignificance?

Meaning and everyday occupation are essentials for life. This is a book that explores the dimensions of meaning in everyday occupation, both the sources of meaning found in occupation and the contributions that occupation makes to meaning in our lives. This is a book about everyday occupation as experience rather than about occupation as task; occupation as experience is occupation as it is perceived through our senses, as it is lived, as it is *experienced*.

In the poem quoted in its entirety above, Adrienne Rich uses the metaphor of a river *delta* to give voice to meanings in her life. The delta is forever changing and deepening, it is the gathering place for the rubble collected by the river along its course, it flows in many directions, and its substance is elusive and difficult to grasp. The delta is the consequence of all the "work" that the river has engaged in as it flows from source to sea. Like the river itself, the delta flows on, spreading its fingers wide as it continues to seek new spheres of being and influence.

Meaning and everyday occupation in our own lives are like the river delta in Adrienne Rich's poem. What we *do* in our day-to-day lives and the meanings created from those doings are inextricably bound together in the flow of life, ever changing and ever deepening, and, yet, at the same time, ever building the delta of our *being*, our *self*, and who we are *becoming*. Each of us has a story that "flows in more than one direction," each of us has "rubble" from our past, and each of us continues to "move on." From an occupational perspective, the everyday occupation of our lives and the meanings of that occupation are essential contributors to the pace and direction of the life flow. Daily occupation may be viewed as the essential current that propels each of us along a lifelong journey. This view of the centrality of occupation to life is reflected in many of the theories of occupation; for example, the theories of the human *need* for occupation as articulated by Wilcock (2006) and the occupational nature of human beings described by Zemke and Clark (1996).

Defining our lives by occupation does not simply mean defining our lives by what we *do*. In addition to the *doing* aspect, occupation offers us experiences of creativity and cultural expression and meaningful connection to the others in our social worlds. Occupation can nurture and release the spiritual aspects of our selves, and, in occupation, we create meaning and significance in the spaces and places in which we live. We will explore these aspects of everyday occupation in the coming chapters of this book.

Throughout the book, verbatim quotations from occupational therapists are used to illustrate and exemplify the concepts being presented and discussed. These quotations are largely drawn from the phenomenological interviews that Virginia Dickie and I conducted with therapists nationwide for our research on the experience of doing occupational therapy (Hasselkus & Dickie, 1994). I also use quotes from other health professionals and family caregivers who participated in some of my other research. Minor details of these quotations are sometimes changed to preserve the anonymity of the research participants and all names are pseudonyms. Finally, I incorporate accounts of my own experiences of everyday occupation into most, if not all, of the chapters. This approach to scholarly writing has been called a "new brand of scholarship that freely mixes personal elements and research expertise" (Heller, 1992). Humanistic geographer Graham Rowles speaks of the power of "interweaving personal experience with scholarly insight" (2008, p. 127). For me, to write authentically about everyday occupational experiences of life requires a personal voice. The feedback I have received from faculty and students since the publication of the first edition in 2002 suggests that the mix of autobiographical elements, verbatim therapy excerpts, and theory and concepts of occupational therapy and occupational science is valued by students and faculty, and it offers strong material for teaching and learning. A new Instructor's Manual, with discussion questions and individual and group activities for each chapter, is available with this edition

New to this revised second edition of *The Meaning of Everyday Occupation* is content on current and developing trends in occupational therapy and occupational science. One such trend is the gradual shifting in our research, education, and practice from an almost exclusive focus on work with individuals to a more encompassing focus on family groups, social communities, and populations as "clients." The increasing need for globalization in the profession is also recognized, in tandem with the inclusion of newly developing cultural concepts such as occupational justice and occupational apartheid. A strengthened emphasis on occupational experiences as transformative processes and recent work on the concept of humans as occupational beings are included. Finally, new theoretical and practice concepts of place integration and therapeutic landscapes are introduced, as are emerging understandings of the field of disability studies and the social and political meanings of disability in the world.

And what of the experience of the reader? Paul Ricoeur, French philosopher of the 20th century, came to believe that to move through life is to navigate a world of texts, each laden with meaning (Fox, 2005). To Ricoeur, the task of human beings is to *interpret* these texts—be they "histories, novels, musical scores, paintings, playscripts, or anything else humans produce that has meaning"—as a way to organize and come to know our world (Vanhoozer, 2005, p. 27). I ask you, the reader, to approach this book with quiet consideration as you seek to read and interpret its text. In Dillard's words, "The reader's ear must adjust down from loud life to the subtle, imaginary sounds of the written word. An ordinary reader picking up a book can't yet hear a thing; it will take half an hour to pick up the writings' modulations, its ups and downs and louds and softs" (1989, p. 17). Reading takes time and imagination, reflection and interpretation; only then can the possibilities for meaningfulness and new understandings of life's deepest experiences be realized.

So I invite you, now, to plunge into the river that awaits you—deeper and deeper into "the heart of the matter," into the meaning and everyday occupation of your life and mine.

# REFERENCES

Dillard, A. (1989). *The writing life.* New York, NY: Harper & Row.

Fox, M. (2005, May 24). Paul Ricoeur, 92, wide-ranging French philosopher, is dead. *New York Times.*

Hasselkus, B. R., & Dickie, V. A. (1994). Doing occupational therapy: Dimensions of satisfaction and dissatisfaction. *American Journal of Occupational Therapy, 48,* 145-154.

Heller, S. (1992, May). Experience and expertise meet in a new brand of scholarship. *The Chronicle of Higher Education,* A7-A9.

Rich, A. (1989). *Time's power.* New York, NY: W. W. Norton & Company, Inc.

Rowles, G. D. (2008). Place in occupational science: A life course perspective on the role of environmental context in the quest for meaning. *Journal of Occupational Science, 15,* 127-135.

Vanhoozer, K. J. (2005, August). The joy of yes. Ricoeur: Philosopher of hope. *Christian Century,* 27-28.

Wilcock, A. A. (2006). *An occupational perspective of health* (2nd ed.). Thorofare, NJ: SLACK Incorporated.

Zemke, R., & Clark, F. (1996). *Occupational science: An evolving discipline.* Philadelphia, PA: F. A. Davis.

# C H A P T E R  1

# MEANING:
# AN ESSENTIAL FOR LIFE

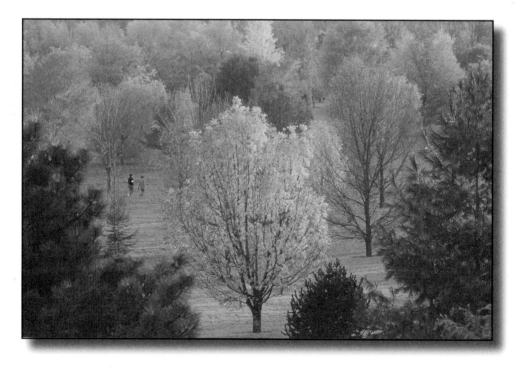

I see the same stars through my window that you see through yours,
But we're worlds apart, worlds apart.

... Together, but worlds apart.

*Big River: The Adventures of Huckleberry Finn*
Miller and Hauptman (1986)

I was born in Wisconsin in the north central part of the United States. I grew up with the night sky of the northern hemisphere—the Big Dipper and Little Dipper, Orion, the North Star, the Milky Way. When I spent several weeks in Australia a few years ago, I eagerly anticipated the new experience of seeing an entirely different array of stars and constellations in the night sky of the southern hemisphere. One night, after dinner at a colleague's home several miles outside of Sydney, my host and the other guests walked outside with me to view the sky; the others, all Australians, helped me "see" this new sky, including, of course, the famed Southern Cross. As we all stood there in the dark, looking up at the stars, in one way we were together, looking at "our" sky from our earth, aware of our shared place in the vastness of the universe and the galaxies beyond. Yet in another way, we were worlds apart. Surely I, seeing this for the first time, was thrilled and moved in ways that were very different from whatever the others were experiencing.

Meaning is largely thought of as an "inside" thing. Meaning does not exist outside the perception and experience of the person within whom it abides. Even when we use language to try to make ideas explicit, meaning remains elusive because, as Polanyi has said, "It is not words that have meaning, but the speaker or listener who means something by them" (1962, p. 252). Polanyi refers to this internal positioning of meaning as the personal mode of meaning; to speak of impersonal meaning is "self-contradictory" (pp. 252-253).

At the same time, however, meaning is public and socially constituted. People's experiences and their meanings are social, "created through interactions," giving them, therefore, "some sort of public status" (Mattingly, 1998, p. 168). Perceptions and experiences are molded by social conventions, beliefs, and attitudes. Iwama (2005) used the term *situated meaning* to describe the importance of cultural context to understandings about meaning for people in the world today and within occupational therapy (p. 127). We are each born into a social world that constitutes who we are—not *all* of who we are, but a significant part of who we are (Benner & Wrubel, 1989). Thus, we may think of meaning as having both shared dimensions and personal dimensions. In meanings, we are together but, also, worlds apart.

Meaning is derived from a person's efforts to make sense out of what he or she is experiencing in day-to-day situations. Making sense out of experiences is a dynamic iterative process of constructing and reconstructing understandings and explanations of everyday living; the "sense" that emerges is part of a "continuing process in which tentative ideas are built upon and elaborated as they are exposed to the exigencies of everyday life" (Hunt, Jordan, & Irwin, 1989, p. 955). Holocaust survivor Frankl stated that the search for meaning is a distinguishing characteristic of being human; we are beings "in steady search of meaning" (1978, p. 20). He viewed this steady search as a "primary motivational force in man," calling it "a will to meaning" (1963, p. 154). In Frankl's view, life never lacks meaning; life is unconditionally meaningful. Medical anthropologist Moerman (2002) agreed, stating, "It is simply not possible to decide to include, or not to include, 'meaning' [in our lives]. It will be there, doing its thing, whether you want it there or not" (p. 130).

Operating on this premise that meaning is present in all of life, I will explore some of the meanings of *meaning* that are offered in the literature. In doing this, I will consider different ways of thinking about meaning as well as ways to gain access to meaning

Hasselkus, B. R.
*The Meaning of Everyday Occupation, Second Edition* (pp. 3-18).
© 2011 SLACK Incorporated

for purposes such as occupational therapy practice and research. I agree with Beer's
statement (1997) that meaning is *real*, despite the fact that it is not accessible to our
usual forms of perception nor can it be described by using scientific methods. Meaning
is real, "*because* it is experienced" (p. 111).

## PERSONAL AND SOCIAL MEANINGS

> The incident I found most dissatisfying occurred during my clinical work as
> a student. A gentleman in his early nineties was referred for ADL [activities
> of daily living] in learning to feed himself. I do not even recall his diagno-
> sis, but I never did understand why he was referred for OT [occupational
> therapy]. From the beginning it was evident that he was not able to respond.
> After several days of therapy, we were notified that the man had died.
> (Hasselkus & Dickie, 1994)

The above quote is a narrative told by a therapist who was asked to think back
over her practice and describe a very dissatisfying experience. One way to describe
this therapist's dissatisfying experience would be to say it was *meaningless* to her; she
"never did understand" why this man was referred to occupational therapy. The German
philosopher Heidegger (1962) would say that an experience may seem meaningless
when the situation is not understandable, is unintelligible. To Heidegger, a sense of
meaninglessness occurs when the possibilities of a situation are not as expected and
the usual meanings have fallen apart. To receive a referral "for ADL" with a patient, and
then to find that patient semi-comatose, flew in the face of all the student had expected
to be able to carry out in therapy. The situation was unintelligible to her. The experience was from her days as a student years before, and yet it remained vividly present
in her memory; of all her practice experiences since then, she chose to describe this
person and this situation in the research interview. The usual, normative meanings of
therapy did not work, they fell apart, and the singular unintelligibility of the situation
became its meaning.

For some of us, meanings in life may be heavily weighted by our personal and
unique values and histories; for others, meanings may stem largely from the community and culture in which we live. From a lifespan perspective, the sources of meaning
in our lives may be thought of as a continuum or as a developmental trajectory that
unfolds throughout life.

### A Continuum of Uniqueness and Community

Reker and Wong (1988) proposed that meaning is situated along a continuum
of contexts, with self-definitions of meaning anchoring one end of the continuum
and social definitions of meaning anchoring the other end. Where a person's sense
of meaning lies along this continuum depends on various factors. For example, the
greater the breadth and depth of experience a person has, the greater will be the contribution of unique personal contexts and history to the meanings in that person's life.
Conversely, a poverty of experiences will yield a person for whom meaning is derived

more strongly from societal expectations. In Reker and Wong's framework, the former person tends toward individualism and the latter toward conformity.

Reker and Wong (1988) implied that the meaning systems of individualists (those on the uniqueness end of the continuum) are better developed, more differentiated than those of conformists. Berman (1993) pointed out that such a view harbors the "Western penchant to view independence, autonomy, and individuality as inherently good" (p. 87). Berman suggested that it may be more helpful to focus instead on the dynamic *interplay* between conformity and individuality that contributes to the creation of meaning throughout life. In Berman's view, life plays out across the lifespan as a never-ending effort to balance our search for uniqueness and self-hood with our search for community and belonging. Meaning in life emanates from this interplay between the two opposing desires.

The student therapist in the above scenario relied heavily on social expectations to make meaning of the situation she was in. At least, it appears that the culturally defined hierarchy within the medical system in which she was functioning (doctor's referral for ADL) and her training in the skills of an occupational therapist (classroom learning about what occupational therapists do) became her definition of "what is" and "what ought to be." She was supposed to carry out the order for ADL with this patient, that's what the doctor told her to do, and that's what occupational therapists are trained to do.

Increasingly, occupational therapy practitioners, researchers, and educators are becoming more aware of the cultural forces that are sometimes invisible but that strongly affect our beliefs and values and actions (Braveman & Bass-Haugen, 2009). These societal forces can lead to health care disparities and injustices and can affect "theory development and proposed interventions regarding the role of occupational therapy" (p. 7). For the student therapist, more experience and perhaps the skills of a mentor might begin to help her understand the situation differently, to see herself in the situation differently, to perceive the situation as one with complex and varied cultural and health care aspects, and to see *possibilities* for meaningful ways of being with this patient. For the student, to be able to see the situation only through the physician's eyes reflects her "frame" to be as others wish her to be. Alternatively, to be able to see the situation in a new and different way (ADL doesn't work here, but touch or music or a scented candle might) would reflect a comfortableness with individualism and uniqueness in an otherwise socially defined circumstance.

## Novice to Expert

Closely related to these lifespan views of meaning is Benner's work on the changing meanings of health care practice across the development of a practitioner's career. Benner (1984), in her book on novice and expert clinical nursing practice, used the term *theoretical knowledge* to describe the knowledge system of the novice nurse clinician and the term *practical knowledge* to describe that of the experienced nurse clinician. Practical knowledge, or "know-how," is developed through the clinical experience of the discipline; according to Benner, experience is "a requisite for expertise" (p. 3). Experience results when "preconceived notions and expectations are challenged, refined, or disconfirmed by the actual situation" (p. 3). Expertise develops when the practitioner recognizes the challenges that are present and subsequently develops and refines the hypotheses and principle-based expectations that are called up in the actual practice situation.

In Benner's model (1984), as the clinician gains experience, his or her clinical performance gradually changes in three general areas: (a) from a reliance on abstract theoretical principles to the use of past personal experience as a guide to practice; (b) from seeing clinical situations as compilations of many bits and pieces to seeing them as wholes in which only certain parts are relevant; and (c) from being in the situation as a detached observer to being an involved performer. Benner's concept of shifting clinical knowledge and performance across time and experience is similar to both Reker and Wong's (1988) concept of a continuum of personal and public meanings and Berman's (1993) focus on the dynamic interplay between conformity and individualism across the lifetime. A person who is inexperienced, such as the student therapist, relies heavily on social definitions of meaning in the situation (theoretical knowledge, norms, principles, socially expected roles); the person who is experienced relies more on his or her personal history to create meaning in the situation, to understand the whole, to become involved. Unfortunately for the student therapist, "experience," as Benner (1984) defined it, did not occur; the student's preconceived notions of what an occupational therapist should do were not challenged or changed by the situation. We know this because, years later, the therapist continues to remember the situation as very dissatisfying, not because she is now aware of other ways in which she could have been with that patient but because she has not, even yet, recognized the challenges, new thinking, and practical knowledge that the situation offered.

## MEANING AND PERFORMANCE IN LIFE

In his writings about the construction and development of the self, Kegan (1982) stated that it is not so much that human beings make meaning in life as it is that the activity of being a person is the activity of meaning-making. "We *are* the meaning making context" (p. 11). To be human is to compose meaning, to make sense. Kegan gives meaning a very active voice; the very act of being a person is an act of meaning making. This action and activity-oriented view of meaning is held by others.

### Meaning as Action

In his book on the meaning found in literature, art, and music, Steiner (1989) argued that to understand and experience aesthetic meaning is to understand and experience the meaning of what it is to be human. Further, it is through *performance* that we enter a life of understanding, because when we perform, we interpret, and interpretation is the source of comprehension. Comprehension enables us to enjoy what Steiner called, "the authentic experience of understanding" (p. 8).

Though Steiner's philosophical discussion was couched in the world of the Arts, and he used the playing of music and the reading of poetry to illustrate the importance of performance to understanding, we may draw parallels to Steiner's views in other realms of life. Steiner (1989) stated that performance is "the action of meaning" (p. 8).

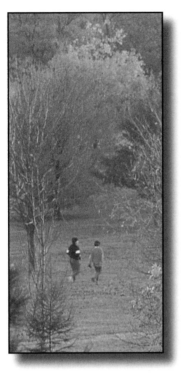

In other words, it is in action or "doing" that meaning is realized in our lives. In the scenario described by the therapist above, I can imagine the frustration and anxiety of the student carrying out prescribed visits to an unresponsive patient for "several days"—confused and frozen by the seeming mismatch between what she was told to do in the referral and the realities of the situation as she perceives it. The expected opportunities to *perform*, to carry out therapy, to be engaged in therapeutic activities were absent. The student found herself in a void—bereft of the usual supports offered by her training.

If we apply Steiner's theory of the intimate connection between authentic understanding in life and performance in life, we could conclude that this void was the natural outcome of the student therapist's perception that there was nothing to *do* with this patient. A more experienced therapist or a therapist who was trained in working with people who are dying might have seen very rich opportunities for performance in this referral, and, in the process of engaging in these opportunities, authentic understandings of the person and the situation might have emerged (Bye, 1998; de Hennezel, 1997; Hasselkus, 1993; Jacques & Hasselkus, 2004). For the experienced therapist, the meaning of the situation might have been the *fullness* of those days.

Recently, in our professional literature, Cutchin (2004) has emphasized to the profession John Dewey's philosophy of active human experience. Cutchin stated that, for Dewey, "situations become the crux of an inquiry into experience and its meaning for individuals or groups" (p. 305). Cutchin introduced the new concept of *place integration* as an authentic representation of the lived experience of human beings in their worlds— proposing an integrated "person-place whole" (p. 310) as a counterpart to the more familiar occupational therapy concepts of person–environment relationships. Cutchin's proposals move our thinking beyond the concepts of "inside" and "outside" and toward thinking of engagement in occupation as a wholeness and oneness of person and place, thus supporting the prominence of *situation* and *context* in meaning-making.

## A Circularity of Constraints

Occupational therapy is a rehabilitative profession that focuses on possibilities for improvement and recovery, independence and health maintenance; the health care system in the United States is heavily oriented toward diagnosing pathology and prescribing a cure. For someone who is dying, such goals do not make sense. For the student therapist, these private and public meanings combined to exert strong constraints on engagement in the situation.

A circularity of constraints may, thus, be set up. To paraphrase Steiner (1989), authentic understandings of a situation emerge through occupational engagement;

without occupational engagement, the ability to develop understandings is constrained. In the former situation, occupational performance leads to unfolding layers of meanings; in the latter situation—the absence of engagement—a person may never be able to perceive the possibilities that lie within the situation, and a sense of emptiness may characterize the experience. Frankl stated that, in finding meaning, "we are perceiving a possibility embedded in reality" (1978, p. 38). If we do not perceive possibilities in a situation, then the potential meanings of the situation lie dormant. Such was the case for the student therapist.

## ASPECTS OF SEEING

Meaning can also be thought of as aspects of seeing. The familiar story of the automobile driver who accidentally backed into a parked car, leaving a sizable dent in the front fender of the other car, comes to mind. In sight of several onlookers, the driver stopped, got out of his car, wrote a note and put it on the windshield of the parked car. All the onlookers saw this action and made the assumption that the man was writing down his name and telephone number so the owner of the other car could contact him. Of course, that is what he hoped they would assume, whereas, in fact, he had written only the words, "Sorry about the fender!" He drove off without anyone taking down his license plate number.

Meaning is related to how we "see" things. This aspect of meaning deserves some discussion.

### *Aspect-Dawning*

*Aspect-dawning* (Wittgenstein, 1968) is the human experience of perceiving not only the outer, informational aspects of objects in a situation or setting (e.g., the behaviors, the shapes, the colors, the textures) but also suddenly perceiving the situation in a different way that is "beyond" the information given by visual observation alone. Suddenly perceiving the action of the man writing the note to be an action different from what was originally thought is an aspect-dawning experience. Once you have "seen" the action as a sham, it is likely that you cannot imagine having *not* seen the note-writing that way before. The meaning of the situation has become clear. The paradox of the aspect-dawning experience is that, once it has occurred, we see the situation differently and yet we also see that the observable aspects of the situation have not changed.

Wittgenstein's (1968) initial descriptions of the aspect-dawning experience were within the context of pictorial symbols, such as drawings and paintings;

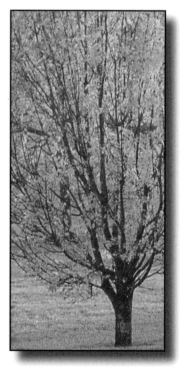

to Wittgenstein, however, the real importance of the experience lay in the fact that the same aspect-dawning experience could occur with written text. In other words (no pun intended), a word is a word is a word—only to a certain extent. The phrase, "That was quite a trip!" could be referring to a spectacular month abroad in France or to a drug-induced state of consciousness; the context would provide cues as to the meaning of the word *trip*. Further, even if we know a priori that the person is writing about a recent vacation in France, the phrase may yet have one of several other kinds of meanings, such as the meaning that the trip was sensational or the meaning that the trip was a disaster. We might misunderstand the meaning at first and then suddenly have an aspect-dawning experience; "Oh! She *hated* it! I thought she meant she *loved* it!" Or we might "get it" right away, in which case the aspect-dawning would occur in immediate response to seeing the words. Thus, Wittgenstein draws this connection between seeing an aspect and experiencing the meaning of words.

Wittgenstein recognized that some people are not able to experience aspect-dawning; he refers to such people as having *aspect-blindness*. Having aspect-blindness does not necessarily mean that the person cannot see an object in more than one way; rather, aspect-blindness means that the person does not feel or *experience* the shift in perception. First the object is this way; then the object is that way. There is no exclamation of "Oh, I thought she meant she loved it!" in spontaneous reaction to the changed perception, as there would be with aspect-dawning. Mulhall (1990) viewed aspect-dawning as a phenomenon that "highlights what is distinctively *human* about human behavior in relation to things in the world, what it is that distinguishes human practical activity from that of automata" (p. 4).

## *Mindfulness*

Somewhat similar to the states of aspect-dawning and aspect-blindness, the concepts of *mindfulness* and *mindlessness* have been proposed by Langer (1989). Langer, too, likened mindfulness to a capacity that enables humans to be more than "automatons" (p. 4). In mindfulness, people welcome and create new information and new categories in their lifeworlds, are aware of many points of view, and focus on process more than outcome in their approach to the routines of the day. Analogous to aspect-blindness, mindlessness is seeing the world in a context-free way. In mindlessness, the events and objects of our worlds are unidimensional; they are what they are regardless of the circumstances that surround their being. In a state of mindlessness, people operate with more automaticity, act from a single perspective, focus on outcome rather than process, and are limited to preset views and labels ("trapped by categories") in their interpretations of daily life (Langer, p. 11).

We might think of the student therapist as having a form of aspect-blindness or mindlessness in the clinical situation with the dying patient. She was unable to act from more than a single perspective, she was unable to "see" the situation in more than one way, her involvement was limited by the preset view that she should be engaging the patient in activities of daily living and there was no way she could do that. She was, in short, trapped by categories—the textbook-like categories that name the rehabilitative ideologies of occupational therapy and thereby constitute what an occupational therapist does in practice. With further experience and input from a mentor, this therapist-in-training might have had her eyes opened to new ways of seeing the situation in a more mindful way—she might have had an aspect-dawning experience about the potential richness of the therapy with someone who is dying. I can almost hear her saying, "Oh, I never thought of it that way!"

## HOW DO WE "KNOW" MEANING?

How do we come to "know" meanings as they occur in our daily lives? Often, we do not know on an explicit level, nor are we able to articulate the meanings of events or relationships in our own lives; how much more difficult, then, it is to know and understand the meanings of events and relationships in other people's lives. And yet, that is what we try to do—as people going about our daily routines in a social world, as occupational therapists in our practice, as researchers studying occupation in people's lives.

Our understandings of the phenomena of our lives are constituted by what MacLachlan and Reid called our "real-world knowledge" (1994, p. 2). Real-world knowledge is built up for each of us across the lifespan as our history of experiences and situations evolves: "It is only by relating new experiences to similar ones from the past that we can begin to make sense of the world" (MacLachlan & Reid, p. 40). Cognitive scientists propose the concept of "knowledge units" or "frames" to capture the way people organize and store this knowledge of everyday experiences (Goffman, 1974; MacLachlan & Reid; Tannen, 1979). People draw upon their frames in any act of interpretation; they "weigh their experiences and expectations" and thereby construct personal meanings of events and phenomena (Hermans, 1989). You, the reader, are drawing on your frames as you read, interpret, and make sense of this text.

Thus, one way to come to understand the meaning of a situation to a person—the way a person frames a situation—is to take the time to learn about the person's life history and past experiences. Out of a person's stories about the past comes the meaning of the present.

### The Narrative Meaning of Therapy

Mattingly (1994, 1998) has offered the concepts of narrative and narrative reasoning to help us understand the storying of life experiences as it occurs in the clinical setting. In narrative theory, people create stories of their life events and experiences as a way to make sense of those events and experiences; by narrativization, people find and create *meaning* in their lives (Bruner, 1986, 1990; Coles, 1989; Kleinman, 1988; Ricoeur,1984). Further, as we create stories of our life events and recount these to others, we are revealing to those others far more than a simple sequence of events: "Events selected, their chronological ordering, and how they are described, contribute to a particular interpretation of events" (Mattingly, 1998, p. 32). In other words, to tell a story is to tell a particular interpretation of an experience. The story of an experience provides a window of understanding into the way the storyteller interprets and frames the events that took place. An understanding of the meaning of the experience may, thus, be gleaned from the story.

Mattingly (1994) proposed that therapists, in each new clinical situation, ask the question: What story am I in? Rather than speaking of treatment goals and plans, Mattingly suggested that therapists speak of prospective stories; that is, of events and experiences that the therapist and client will create as they weave a new story together. In our research on the meaning of doing occupational therapy (Hasselkus & Dickie, 1994), Virginia Dickie suggested the metaphor of a *moiré* to describe the end result of this storying together. The word *moiré* refers to a new pattern that is created when two previously separate patterns are superimposed on each other. In the context of meaning and therapy, the therapist's and client's individual stories become superimposed on each other and a new communal story is created. Put another way, the therapist and the client each bring their own real-world knowledge—their histories and ways of framing life—to the therapy situation. If the histories are shared and the frames are superimposed on each other, a new shared story emerges as the therapy unfolds.

Narratives as sources of meaning thus offer a way for us to frame the practice of occupational therapy. Therapy can be viewed not only as an event in which the therapist enters the story of the client (Helfrich & Kielhofner, 1994) but also as one in which a client enters the story (world) of the therapist (Rosa & Hasselkus, 2005).

Yet, whether or not an occupational therapist actually uses a narrative metaphor to describe practice, he or she can develop and use strategies designed specifically to gain understanding of clients' ways of framing their life experiences (Crepeau, 1991; Frank, Huecker, Segal, Forwell, & Bagatell, 1991; Helfrich & Kielhofner, 1994; Mallinson, Kielhofner, & Mattingly, 1996; Rosa & Hasselkus, 2005; Schön, 1983). Ethnographic interviewing techniques can be used during therapist–client interactions to gain understanding of the client's life perspective (Hasselkus, 1990; Spencer, Krefting, & Mattingly, 1993). As Peloquin (1993) has stated, "illness and disability are events charged with personal meaning" (p. 830). Without a therapeutic approach that recognizes the need to come to understand those personal meanings, the therapist may be perceived by the client as distant, brusque, and discouraging; as withholding information and feelings; and as misusing power (Peloquin). *With* a therapeutic approach that incorporates time and strategies to gain understanding of the client's history and story and to share the therapist's story with the client, a moiré can be created—a new story that fits the fundamental beliefs and values of both client and therapist.

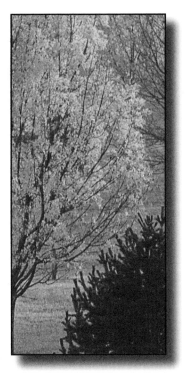

## *Interpretive Research*

Research approaches to the discovery and understanding of meaning in our lives are richly varied. In trying to describe and articulate invisible, unobservable phenomena such as meaning, various schemata have been proposed.

Many research traditions such as grounded theory, life history, phenomenology, and ethnography rely on the expression of "ordinary language" for data. Narrative storytelling, reviews of life documents, participant observation, and interpretive interviewing are data collection strategies that may be represented in all of these traditions. In occupational therapy, the ground-breaking ethnographic research on clinical reasoning by Mattingly and Fleming (1994) led to an initial predilection for ethnography as the choice for interpretive research on occupation within the field. More recently, institutional ethnography, autoethnography, life history, and phenomenology have been emerging in the occupational therapy research literature as well (Dickie, 1997; Frank, 1996, 2000; Hasselkus & Murray, 2007; Johansson & Tham, 2006; Neville-Jan, 2003; Townsend, Langille, & Ripley, 2003). As an example, Johansson and Tham used phenomenology to study the experience of work after acquired brain injury; their stated purpose was to gain understanding of "the meaning structure of the phenomenon under study" (p. 61).

Narrative as a construction of meaning offers us one way to frame our research about meaning and occupation. In Polkinghorne's (1988) book on narrative knowing, he made the following statement: "According to a narrative theory of human experience, a study needs to focus its attention on existence as it is lived, experienced, and interpreted by the human person" (p. 125). In Polkinghorne's view, research into meaning requires the use of linguistic expression and thinking processes such as analogy and pattern recognition. Because meaning is not directly observable, it must be approached through self-reflection and introspection. Also, in this view, because meaning is not a material thing, understanding of meaning is "best captured through the qualitative nuances of its expression in ordinary languages" (p. 10).

## Objectified Research

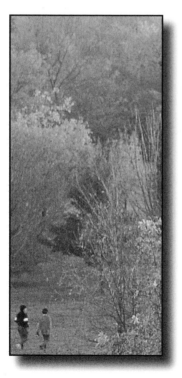

Another tradition of research on meaning and occupation is represented by the use of quantitative or experimental approaches to study meaning. Research that uses Osgood's Meaning Differential (Osgood, Suci, & Tannenbaum, 1957), a standardized paper-and-pencil instrument for measuring meaning in activities, is represented in the early work of Nelson and his associates (Adelstein & Nelson, 1985; Nelson, 1988; Rocker & Nelson, 1987). From this work, Nelson formulated his concepts of occupational form, occupational performance, and therapeutic occupation (Nelson, 1988, 1996). In 1988, Nelson defined occupational form as the objective set of circumstances external to the person (i.e., the context) that elicits, guides, and structures human performance; *meaning*, in this formulation, refers to "the individual's interpretation of the occupational form" (p. 635). In 1996, Nelson expanded on this definition of meaning, adding the following: "Meaning is the sense that the person makes of a situation"; further, meaning includes "perceptual, symbolic, and affective experience" (Nelson, 1996, p. 776). Nelson linked meaning to purpose in his definitions, saying that, after a person finds meaning in a situation, "he or she experiences purpose, or the desire to do something about the situation" (1996, p. 777).

Trombly (1995) extended this thinking about purpose and meaning further. To Trombly, purposefulness *organizes* our time and behavior, and *meaningfulness* motivates our performance in occupation. Ferguson and Trombly (1997) tried to operationally separate purposefulness from meaningfulness and to study how each was related to scores on a motor learning task. In their findings, participation by subjects in an added-purpose occupation resulted in significantly greater motor learning than participation in a rote exercise; scores were not related, however, to the level of meaning (on an analog scale from high to low) assigned to the occupation. The authors stated in their conclusions that, in their attempt to tease apart the two phenomena of purpose and meaning, they had little control over the type and level of meaning that subjects assigned to the two conditions. The impact of meaning remained elusive since it depended on "the level of interest, importance, value, and so forth that the subject held for the activity" (Ferguson & Trombly, p. 513).

## *Mix and Match*

Using a combination of narrative and quantitative data, social psychologist Csikszentmihalyi (1990) developed the experience sampling method (ESM) of data collection to study the meaning of daily activity. Subjects in his research carried a beeper or programmed wristwatch and were beeped at random intervals throughout the day; upon being beeped, each participant filled out a standard form that addressed questions about what the person was doing at the time of the signal, what his or her sense of control was, and what degree of challenge was present at the time. Out of this research, Csikszentmihalyi generated his concept of *flow*, a term to describe the subjective quality of engagement in daily occupations. Although developed within the discipline of psychology, the ESM has been used and continues to be used by occupational therapists to study the meaning of the experience of occupation (Jacobs, 1994; Kennedy, 1998; Larson & von Eye, 2010; Toth-Fejel, Toth-Fejel, & Hedricks, 1998).

Other research that mixes qualitative and quantitative research questions and methods is also being generated by scholars within the field. Dickie and her co-researchers carried out a qualitative study focusing on parents' reports of sensory experiences in preschool children with and without autism (Dickie, Baranek, Schultz, Watson, & McComish, 2009). The narrative data generated by the participating parents constituted one component of an ongoing quantitative study of hyper-responsiveness in children with autism, developmental delay, and typical development. Dickie et al. felt that the qualitative component of the study added a "unique and personal perspective of sensory experiences in the children's daily functioning" (p. 180). The study by Dickie et al. represents an effort to understand the meanings ascribed to the children's sensory experiences by the parents, using narrative data to generate those understandings.

# THE OPEN DOOR POLICY

So where does this take us? Trying to understand a phenomenon that cannot be seen puzzles us. Bruner (1986) felt that to understand the unseen requires a different way of thinking. He conceptualized human beings as having two modes of thought—the logico-scientific mode and the narrative mode. The former represents our formal, mathematical system of description and explanation; the narrative mode, alternatively, houses the imagination, consciousness, the particulars of experience, and concern for the human condition. To Bruner, it is in the narrative mode that life and its experiences can be known.

Heidegger (1966) also denoted two modes of human thought, calling them *calculative thinking* and *meditative thinking*: "Calculative thinking computes … [it] is the mark of all thinking that plans and investigates." Meditative thinking is that "which contemplates the meaning which reigns in everything that is" (p. 46). Expanding on the concept of meditative thinking, Van Manen (1997) suggested that there are two modes of meaning—thematic meaning and expressive meaning. *Thematic meaning* is drawn from the informational content of a phenomenon, and *expressive meaning* is more an "inner" grasping of the poetic, the situational, the nontheoretical aspects of the phenomenon. Van Manen suggested that thematic meanings are cognitive, designative, and particular; expressive meanings go beyond cognition to illuminate the emotive spirit of phenomena.

The narrative mode, the meditative mode, and expressive meaning are proposed as the ways of being-in-the-world that have "the power to break through the taken-for-granted dimensions of everyday life" (Van Manen, 1997, p. 346). They are the products of our conclusions that to understand meaning requires modes of thought and expression that are different from our everyday purposeful ways of thinking. To overcome these rather dichotomizing concepts, Belenky, Clinchy, Goldberger, and Tarule (1986) described an *integrative* way of knowing in which intuitive knowledge is integrated with knowledge gained from the external world. In their study of women's ways of knowing, one participant said that, in integrated thinking, "You let the inside out and the outside in" (p. 135). Integrative thought weaves together "strands of rational and emotive thought … of objective and subjective knowing" (p. 134). In other words, to think integratively about the meanings of the phenomena of our world, we must first open the door so that we can "let the inside out and the outside in"; we must accept and experience the world as *possibilities* and ourselves as able to *live* in possibilities (Heidegger, 1962). Only then might we finally grasp the whole of this elusive concept of meaning in our lives.

… Together, but worlds apart.

# REFERENCES

Adelstein, L. A., & Nelson, D. L. (1985). Effects of sharing versus non-sharing on affective meaning in collage activities. *Occupational Therapy in Mental Health, 5,* 29-45.

Beer, D. W. (1997). "There's a certain Slant of light": The experience of discovery in qualitative interviewing. *Occupational Therapy Journal of Research, 17,* 110-129.

Belenky, M. F., Clinchy, B. M., Goldberger, N. R., & Tarule, J. M. (1986). *Women's ways of knowing: The development of self, voice, and mind.* New York, NY: Basic Books.

Benner, P. (1984). *From novice to expert.* Menlo Park, CA: Addison-Wesley.

Benner, P., & Wrubel, J. (1989). *The primacy of caring: Stress and coping in health and illness.* Menlo Park, CA: Addison-Wesley.

Berman, H. J. (1993). The tree and the vine: Existential meaning and Olmstead's personal journal of retirement. *Journal of Aging Studies, 7,* 81-92.

Braveman, B., & Bass-Haugen, J. D. (2009). Social justice and health disparities: An evolving discourse in occupational therapy research and intervention. *American Journal of Occupational Therapy, 63,* 7-12.

Bruner, J. (1986). *Actual minds. Possible worlds.* Cambridge, MA: Harvard University Press.

Bruner, J. (1990). *Acts of meaning.* Cambridge, MA: Harvard University Press.

Bye, R. A. (1998). When clients are dying: Occupational therapists' perspectives. *Occupational Therapy Journal of Research, 18,* 3-24.

Coles, R. (1989). *The call of stories.* Cambridge, MA: Harvard University Press.

Crepeau, E. B. (1991). Achieving intersubjective understanding: Examples from an occupational therapy session. *American Journal of Occupational Therapy, 45,* 1016-1025.

Csikszentmihalyi, M. (1990). *Flow: The psychology of optimal experience.* New York, NY: Harper & Row.

Cutchin, M. P. (2004). Using Deweyan philosophy to rename and reframe adaptation-to-environment. *American Journal of Occupational Therapy, 58,* 303-312.

de Hennezel, M. (1997). *Intimate death: How the dying teach us how to live.* New York, NY: Alfred A. Knopf.

Dickie, V. (1997). Insights from a focused autobiography. *Occupational Therapy Journal of Research, 17,* 99-104.

Dickie, V. A., Baranek, G. T., Schultz, B., Watson, L. R., & McComish, C. S. (2009). Parent reports of sensory experiences of preschool children with and without autism: A qualitative study. *American Journal of Occupational Therapy, 63,* 172-181.

Ferguson, J. M., & Trombly, C. A. (1997). Effect of added-purpose and meaningful occupation on motor learning. *American Journal of Occupational Therapy, 51,* 508-515.

Frank, G. (1996). Life histories in occupational therapy clinical practice. *American Journal of Occupational Therapy, 50,* 251-264.

Frank, G. (2000). *Venus on wheels: Two decades of dialogue on disability, biography, and being female in America.* Berkeley, CA: University of California Press.

Frank, G., Huecker, E., Segal, R., Forwell, S., & Bagatell, N. (1991). Assessment and treatment of a pediatric patient in chronic care: Ethnographic methods applied to occupational therapy practice. *American Journal of Occupational Therapy, 45,* 252-263.

Frankl, V. E. (1963). *Man's search for meaning.* New York, NY: Washington Square Press.

Frankl, V. E. (1978). *The unheard cry for meaning.* New York, NY: Simon and Schuster.

Goffman, E. (1974). *Frame analysis: An essay on the organization of experience.* Cambridge, MA: Harvard University Press.

Hasselkus, B. R. (1990). Ethnographic interviewing: A tool for practice with family caregivers for the elderly. *Occupational Therapy Practice, 2,* 9-16.

Hasselkus, B. R. (1993). Death in very old age: A personal journey of caregiving. *American Journal of Occupational Therapy, 47,* 717-723.

Hasselkus, B. R., & Dickie, V. A. (1994). Doing occupational therapy: Dimensions of satisfaction and dissatisfaction. *American Journal of Occupational Therapy, 48,* 145-154.

Hasselkus, B. R., & Murray, B. J. (2007). Everyday occupation, well-being and identity: The experience of caregivers in families with dementia. *American Journal of Occupational Therapy, 61,* 9-20.

Heidegger, M. (1962). *Being and time.* (Macquarrie & Robinson, Trans.). San Francisco, CA: Harper Collins.

Heidegger, M. (1966). *Discourse on thinking.* New York, NY: Harper & Row.

Helfrich, C., & Kielhofner, G. (1994). Volitional narratives and the meaning of therapy. *American Journal of Occupational Therapy, 48,* 319-326.

Hermans, H. J. M. (1989). The meaning of life as an organized process. *Psychotherapy, 26,* 11-22.

Hunt, L. M., Jordan, B., & Irwin, S. (1989). Views of what's wrong: Diagnosis and patients' concepts of illness. *Social Science & Medicine, 28,* 945-956.

Iwama, M. K. (2005). Situated meaning: An issue of culture, inclusion, and occupational therapy. In F. Kronenberg, S. S. Algado, & N. Pollard (Eds.), *Occupational therapy without borders* (pp. 127-139). New York, NY: Elsevier Limited.

Jacobs, K. (1994). Flow and the occupational therapy practitioner. *American Journal of Occupational Therapy, 48,* 989-996.

Jacques, N., & Hasselkus, B. R. (2004). The nature of occupation surrounding dying and death. *OTJR: Occupation, Participation and Health, 24,* 44-53.

Johansson, U., & Tham, K. (2006). The meaning of work after acquired brain injury. *American Journal of Occupational Therapy, 60,* 60-69.

Kegan, R. (1982). *The evolving self.* Cambridge, MA: Harvard University Press.

Kennedy, B. L. (1998). *Feeling and doing: Health and mind-body-context interactions during daily occupations of women with HIV/AIDS.* Unpublished doctoral dissertation, University of Southern California, Ann Arbor, MI.

Kleinman, A. (1988). *The illness narratives.* New York, NY: Basic Books.

Langer, E. J. (1989). *Mindfulness.* New York, NY: Addison-Wesley.

Larson, E., & von Eye, A. (2010). Beyond flow: Temporality and participation in everyday activities. *American Journal of Occupational Therapy, 64,* 152-163.

MacLachlan, G., & Reid, I. (1994). *Framing and interpretation.* Melbourne, Australia: Melbourne University Press.

Mallinson, T., Kielhofner, G., & Mattingly, C. (1996). Metaphor and meaning in a clinical interview. *American Journal of Occupational Therapy, 50,* 338-346.

Mattingly, C. (1994). The narrative nature of clinical reasoning. In C. Mattingly & M. H. Fleming (Eds.), *Clinical reasoning: Forms of inquiry in a therapeutic practice* (pp. 239-269). Philadelphia, PA: F. A. Davis.

Mattingly, C. (1998). *Healing dramas and clinical plots: The narrative structure of experience.* Cambridge, UK: Cambridge University Press.

Mattingly, C., & Fleming, M. (1994). *Clinical reasoning: Forms of inquiry in a therapeutic practice.* Philadelphia, PA: F. A. Davis.

Miller, R., & Hauptman, W. (composer). (1986). *Big river: The adventures of Huckleberry Finn.* (1st Grove Press ed.). New York, NY: Grove Press.

Moerman, D. (2002). *Meaning, medicine and the "placebo effect."* Cambridge, UK: Cambridge University Press.

Mulhall, S. (1990). *On being in the world.* New York, NY: Routledge.

Nelson, D. L. (1988). Occupation: Form and performance. *American Journal of Occupational Therapy, 42,* 633-641.

Nelson, D. L. (1996). Therapeutic occupation: A definition. *American Journal of Occupational Therapy, 50,* 775-782.

Neville-Jan, A. (2003). Encounters in a world of pain: An autoethnography. *American Journal of Occupational Therapy, 57,* 88-98.

Osgood, C. E., Suci, G. J., & Tannenbaum, P. H. (1957). *The measurement of meaning.* Urbana, IL: University of Illinois Press.

Peloquin, S. M. (1993). The depersonalization of patients: A profile gleaned from narratives. *American Journal of Occupational Therapy, 47,* 830-837.

Polanyi, M. (1962). *Personal knowledge: Towards a post-critical philosophy.* Chicago, IL: University of Chicago Press.

Polkinghorne, D. E. (1988). *Narrative knowing and the human sciences.* Albany, NY: SUNY Press.

Reker, G. T., & Wong, P. T. P. (1988). Aging as an individual process: Toward a theory of personal meaning. In J. E. Birren & V. L. Bengtson (Eds.), *Emergent theories of aging* (pp. 214-246). New York, NY: Springer.

Ricoeur, P. (1984). *Time and narrative.* Chicago, IL: University of Chicago Press.

Rocker, J. D., & Nelson, D. L. (1987). Affective responses to keeping or not keeping an activity product. *American Journal of Occupational Therapy, 41,* 152-157.

Rosa, S., & Hasselkus, B. R. (2005). Finding common ground with patients: The centrality of compatibility. *American Journal of Occupational Therapy, 59,* 198-208.

Schön, D. A. (1983). *The reflective practitioner: How professionals think in action.* New York, NY: Basic Books.

Spencer, J., Krefting, L., & Mattingly, C. (1993). Incorporation of ethnographic methods in occupational therapy assessment. *American Journal of Occupational Therapy, 47,* 303-309.

Steiner, G. (1989). *Real presences.* Chicago, IL: University of Chicago Press.

Tannen, D. (1979). What's in a frame? Surface evidence for underlying expectations. In R. O. Freedle (Ed.), *New directions in discourse processing* (pp. 137-181). Norwood, NJ: Ablex.

Toth-Fejel, G. E., Toth-Fejel, G. F., & Hedricks, C. A. (1998). Occupation-centered practice in hand rehabilitation using the experience sampling method. *American Journal of Occupational Therapy, 52,* 381-385.

Townsend, E., Langille, L., & Ripley, D. (2003). Professional tensions in client-centered practice: Using institutional ethnography to generate understanding and transformation. *American Journal of Occupational Therapy, 57,* 17-28.

Trombly, C. A. (1995). Occupation, purposefulness and meaningfulness as therapeutic mechanisms. *American Journal of Occupational Therapy, 49,* 960-972.

Van Manen, M. (1997). From meaning to method. *Qualitative Health Research 7,* 345-369.

Wittgenstein, L. (1968). *Philosophical investigations* (G. E. M. Anscombe, Trans.). Oxford, UK: Basil Blackwell.

# CHAPTER 2

# MEANING IN EVERYDAY OCCUPATION

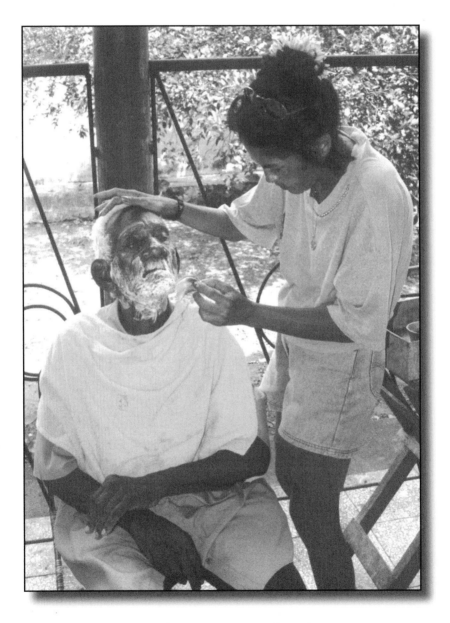

The nature of humans is to make meaning through occupation.

Crabtree (1998, p. 205)

In the Introduction to this book, I drew from Adrienne Rich's poem "Delta" to create a metaphor of life as a flowing river—ever moving on, ever changing, ever expanding into more and more channels, ever creating and re-creating itself. As part of the metaphor, I described daily occupation as "the essential current that propels each of us along" on life's journey; "… the occupations of our lives and the meanings of those occupations are essential contributors to the pace and direction of the life flow."

In this chapter, I explore the relationship between meaning and occupation. Occupation is a powerful source of meaning in our lives; meaning arises from occupation and occupation arises from meaning. Crabtree (1998), as quoted on p. 20, stated that it is the nature of humans to make meaning through occupation; yet, it is also possible to turn this statement around and say that it is the nature of humans to create occupation from meanings. Either way, occupation and meaning are inextricably intertwined in our lives, each contributing to the other throughout our life spans.

The bioethicist and philosopher Engelhardt (1983) has stated that occupational therapists are meaning-givers. According to Engelhardt, the English word *therapy* is derived from a Greek word for "wooing" or "courting." He argued that, as therapy personnel, we do not simply engage in technical procedures. Rather, we engage in a process of wooing as we work with clients to help them understand their situations and the purposes of the therapy we are trying to carry out. In Engelhardt's words, we are, in effect, "wooing meaning" (p. 141), for, as he further states, "it is only within a context of meaning that treatment can take place" (p. 142).

In creating a context of meaning, we are both wooers of meaning and meaning-givers; we seek to elicit and discover the meanings of the situation and we offer occupation as a way to respond to those meanings and to help create new meaning. Thought of in this way, occupation becomes, by definition, the vehicle for creating meaning in the occupational therapy context of care, and occupational therapists become, as Engelhardt has said, custodians of meaning.

# HAPPINESS IS ...

My last job was at a skilled nursing facility in a small state hospital. What stands out in my mind was one gentleman who was a post CVA [cerebrovascular accident] with a very contracted left arm. He had been dominantly right handed, so he was still capable of doing very much with his right hand. However, no one really took the time, prior to my coming there, to work with him and find out what his interests were and just how he could gain back his self-esteem and his abilities again to function as a happy man, not a disgruntled man.

He liked to do small craft work; he had done some carving and whittling prior to his CVA as a pastime. So I rigged up a little contraption, a little wooden form with some vises that would hold things for him, and little bit by little bit—he was a little apprehensive at first—we did get some tools for him and eventually I did work with him and get him into a line of productivity that made him very happy. And we had him look forward to getting up in the morning.

Hasselkus, B. R.
*The Meaning of Everyday Occupation, Second Edition* (pp. 21-38).
© 2011 SLACK Incorporated

So in the end, we made this man a very happy man … because he had been very, so very unhappy for such a long time … But he was very happy that he was able to be productive again and, indeed, [it] gave him self-esteem, and he became a much more liked man on the unit with everyone that came in contact with him. And we have pictures of him with his craftwork. So, that's the man that stands out best in my mind that I have always felt I accomplished a lot with.

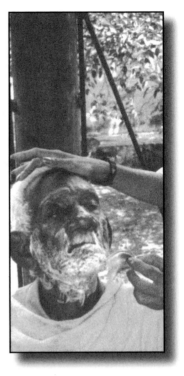

The experience above was described by an occupational therapist who participated in a research study on the meaning of doing occupational therapy (Hasselkus & Dickie, 1994). The story was the therapist's response to the researcher's request to "Think back over your practice and describe a very satisfying experience." The story is one of using occupation to help a person move from a state of ill-being ("so very unhappy for such a long time") to a state of well-being ("a very happy man," "a much more liked man"). In keeping with Engelhardt (1983), the therapist described a situation in which she did much more than engage in technical procedures. She helped to build meaningfulness back into the daily life of this man; she was a meaning-giver. In the therapist's view, these were accomplishments that far outweighed this man's regained ability to carve and whittle. Not one mention is made in the story, even in its entirety, about *what* the man carved; rather, the emphasis is on the changes that occurred in his mood and his outlook on life and how he was perceived by others.

## Defining Occupation

In our profession, we have struggled in recent decades to define *occupation* and to promote the centrality of the concept in occupational therapy (American Occupational Therapy Association [AOTA], 1993, 1995, 2008; Canadian Association of Occupational Therapy [CAOT], 1997, 2002; Clark et al., 1991; Golledge, 1998; Nelson, 1996; Parham, 1998; Pierce, 2001; Trombly, 1995; Yerxa, 1994; Zemke & Clark, 1996). Clark et al. posed an early definition of occupation as "the ordinary and familiar things that people do every day" (p. 300). Yerxa expanded the definition, stating that occupation is "engagement in self-initiated, self-directed, adaptive, purposeful, culturally relevant, organized activity" (p. 587). In 1996, Zemke and Clark brought forward the somewhat awkward definition of occupation as "chunks of daily activity that can be named in the lexicon of the culture" (p. vii). More comprehensive, but also cumbersome, is the definition proposed by Law, Polatajko, Baptiste, and Townsend in 1997:

> Occupation refers to groups of activities and tasks of everyday life, named, organized, and given value and meaning by individuals and a culture. Occupation is everything people do to occupy themselves, including looking

after themselves (self-care), enjoying life (leisure), and contributing to the social and economic fabric of their communities (productivity). (p. 34)

In 1998, Golledge once again simplified the definition by proposing that occupation be defined as "the daily living tasks that are part of an individual's lifestyle" (p. 102).

In 2001, Pierce plowed new ground as she made an effort to "untangle" the concepts of occupation and activity. Her primary distinction between the two terms seems to be that occupation is the subjective experience of an individual, with meaning that is personally constructed; activity, on the other hand, is a culturally defined class of human actions, shared in the minds and cultural language of persons. For example, by Pierce's definitions, the Monopoly game that a family plays together one evening is one kind of occupation (a personal subjective experience), but the idea of board games with their rules, turn-taking, winning and losing, moving pieces about the board, bonuses and penalties, etc., is an activity (culturally defined and shared). Finally, most recently, AOTA's second edition of the *Occupational Therapy Practice Framework* (2008) skirts the problem of trying to provide one definition by simply listing six different definitions found in the literature.

## Shifting Trends

In very recent years, a movement has emerged within the profession that calls for the broadening of definitions of occupation beyond the historical (and almost exclusive) focus on the *individual* client to a view of occupation that also reflects *interdependence* and *community* (AOTA, 2008; Dickie, Cutchin, & Humphry, 2006; Hammell, 2009a; Iwama, 2005; Watson, 2004). Hammell (2009a) reminded us that values of individualism and independence are not universal values in our world; they reflect specific Western ideologies, and are not present in majority-world cultures that value "reciprocal obligations and harmonious relationships" (p. 10). Dickie et al (2006) also argued that the profession is not served well by definitions of occupation that focus "almost entirely on individual experience" (p. 83). Reflecting this thinking, more and more occupational science research and publications demonstrate the application of principles of occupation and health beyond individual clients to larger units of families, communities, and populations in the world (Bonder, 2006; DeGrace, 2003; Kronenberg, Algado, & Pollard, 2005; Watson & Swartz, 2004). Social concepts such as occupational deprivation, occupational injustice, and occupational apartheid are being formulated and discussed (Kronenberg et al., 2005; Townsend & Wilcock, 2004); recognition of meaningful and purposeful occupation as a universal right of all people is gaining attention (Hammell, 2008; Watson & Fourie, 2004). A global view of the profession, with awareness of social justice issues and health disparities, is gradually being realized (Blakeney & Marshall, 2009; Braveman & Bass-Haugen, 2009).

A second shift in professional thinking is represented in efforts to reexamine the basic categories of self-care, leisure, and work that have long been used to define and describe the essence of occupation (Dickie, 2009; Hammell, 2009a, 2009b; Hasselkus, 2006; Jonsson, 2008; Primeau, 1998). Hammell referred to these categories as "simplistic" and "arbitrary" (2009b, p. 107), and Dickie stated that the categories are "often problematic," citing the example that what is leisure for one person may be work for another, or what a person experiences as leisure on one day may be experienced—by the same person—as work on another (p. 19). One response to this emerging shift away from the model of three broad categories has been to retain the focus on *kinds* of occupation but to divide it into more discrete categories. The *AOTA Occupational Therapy Practice Framework* (2008) divides occupation into "areas" as follows: "activities of daily living, instrumental activities of daily living, rest and sleep, education, work, play, leisure, and social participation" (p. 630). All areas are then further broken down into a comprehensive total listing of 42 "life activities" (pp. 631–633). In a different response, Hammell (2009) proposes, "Instead of being categorized as self-care, productivity, and leisure, research findings suggest that occupation could more usefully be categorized according to people's *experiences* of occupational engagement" (p. 113, emphasis added). Jonsson also suggested experience-based categories of occupation such as "relaxing," "engaging," and "time-killing" (p. 6).

The effort to reach consensus on the meaning and definition of occupation continues. Perhaps, as Dickie stated, "The construct of occupation might very well defy efforts to reduce it to a single definition or a set of categories" (2009, p. 19). Nevertheless, read on …

## Breaking Out of the Box

Many of these definitions, as can be readily seen, focus heavily on occupation as "doing." They incorporate words of action, engagement, personal initiative, purposefulness, activity, and tasks; they refer to what people "do." In the spring of 1998, at the World Federation of Occupational Therapists Congress, Montréal, Canada, Ann Wilcock broke out of this "box" in her keynote address by describing occupation as "the synthesis of doing, being, and becoming" (1998a, p. 249; 1998b). I was in the audience on that day, and I found myself captivated by her thinking. The doing of occupation was not discarded, but being and becoming were added. In Wilcock's view, doing, being, and becoming were "integral to occupational therapy philosophy, process, and outcomes, because together they epitomize occupation" (p. 249). Our sense of who we *are* as human beings and who we *are becoming* contributes to the intelligibility of our lives. Our being and our becoming are part of our life stories as they are lived and created anew each day; being and becoming emanate from the everyday doing of our lives.

Three years later, expanding beyond Wilcock's three dimensions of occupation, Rebeiro and her colleagues identified themes of being, becoming, and *belonging* as major health needs of participants in a community mental health program (Rebeiro, Day, Semeniuk, O'Brien, & Wilson, 2001). In 2004, Hammell probed more deeply into what she referred to as the "dimensions of meaning" (p. 296) in daily occupations, including all four themes—doing, being, belonging, and becoming. Hammell suggested, at that time, that a focus on meaning might be the best way to understand the concept of occupation. And now, in the second edition of her book, Wilcock has added the dimension of belonging to her thinking, proposing a model of occupation as "doing + being, becoming, belonging = survival and health" (2006, p. 220).

We can use these four dimensions of occupation to interpret the therapist's story about the man whom she enabled to resume his hobbies of whittling and carving. The doing part of the story is perhaps obvious—the therapist "rigged up a little contraption" and got him some tools and worked with him until she was able to "get him into a line of productivity that made him very happy." But as I stated earlier, in her story, the therapist did not actually name any of the items that the man had carved. Instead, she described his *being*: "We made this man a very happy man" and "gave him self-esteem." Previously, his *being* had been as a disgruntled man who was "so very unhappy." The *becoming* of the man is also evident in the story; change is described in the statement that "he was a little apprehensive at first" and the therapist "did work with him" and eventually "we had him look forward to getting up in the morning." Looking forward to getting up in the morning is another way of saying that *becoming* is part of a person's life—each new day is looked forward to, possibilities are understood, meaningfulness is present. And finally, the dimension of *belonging* is revealed in the therapist's statement that "he became a much more liked man *on the unit* with *everyone* that came in contact with him" (emphasis added). The importance of relationships and social context and being a part of a larger community is acknowledged in this therapist's description of the man and his occupation. Occupation as a synthesis of doing, being, becoming, and belonging is a good fit with this occupational narrative.

In a way, these four dimensions of occupation represent yet another artificial division of occupation into parts—different from dividing occupation into self-care, leisure, and work but a division nonetheless. And as soon as we try to focus on any one part—the doing, being, becoming, or belonging—an awkwardness immediately surfaces, for the four are intertwined. Nevertheless, for the purpose of increased understanding of meaning and occupation, for the rest of this chapter I will endeavor to delve more deeply into the dimensions that, to me, at this point in time, best represent meaning—being, becoming, and belonging.

## OCCUPATION AND BEING

Parker Palmer (2000), in his small book about discovering one's path in life, makes the following statement about the human self and its potential: "Our deepest calling is to grow into our own authentic selfhood. ... As we do so, we will not only find the joy that every human being seeks—we will also find our path of authentic service in the world" (p. 16). This is Palmer's passionate message: To know one's self is both to know the world and to know one's authentic path within that world.

### To Know One's Self

Occupation is a strong enabler for knowing one's self. To know one's self is to know one's *being*. One way that my self becomes known to me is through occupation and one way that my self expresses itself in the world is through occupation. Occupation helps me answer questions such as: What am I meant to do? Who am I meant to be? Is the life I am living authentic? Am I growing into my authentic selfhood? Is the life I am living the same as the life that wants to live in me? (Palmer, 2000, p. 2).

From a related but somewhat different perspective, Christiansen, in his 1999 Eleanor Clark Slagle Lecture, presented a view of occupation as "the principal means through which people develop and express their personal identities" (p. 547). To begin examining this proposed theory, DeGroat, Lyons, and Tickle-Degnen (2006) conducted an exploratory study of the relationship of occupation to identity in people with Parkinson's disease and found that "cues about personality and mood, in addition to the occupational preferences of clients ... learned during client interviews, can give practitioners clearer insight into the personal identity of occupational therapy clients" (p. 66). Although identity is not the same as selfhood, it is one form of expression of the self. The shaping of one's identity by occupation and experience has been called *selfing* (McAdams, 1997)—that is, "the process of being a self" (p. 56). McAdams stated that the greater the number and variety of life possibilities, the greater the uncertainty about what an integrated "me" should look like, and the greater the challenge that is experienced as people try to forge selves that are unified and purposeful. Selfing puts human experiences together, synthesizes them, and unifies them, so that they are thought of as one's own, as phenomena that "belong to me," that are "mine." Identity is the product of this selfing process; identity is the expression of one's unified being and purpose in life. Occupation is a principal agent in the selfing process that helps forge identity.

The concepts of *self* and *identity* are closely related to each other and to the concept of being. Kegan (1982), in his provocative book on the developing self referred to in chapter 1, has stated that it is not that a person *makes* meaning, but, rather, that "Human being is the composing of meaning" (p. 11). In other words, we humans *are* meaning-making. Kegan referred to a person's self as "the zone of mediation where meaning is made" (p. 3). For each of us, our self is the place "between an event and a reaction to it—the place where the event is privately composed, made sense of, the place where it actually *becomes* an event" for us (p. 2). The self is the place where meaning is made of our world and of our engagement in that world.

## Let Your Life Speak or Set Goals?

Palmer (2000) believes that we are born into this life with an inner being that is ready to unfold as a guiding path in our lives. This path is what Palmer calls our "way" or our "vocation." Palmer's message is in the title and subtitle of his book, *Let Your Life Speak: Listening for the Voice of Vocation.* In other words, our way, our being, our vocation is present within us, "not as a goal to be achieved but as a gift to be received" (p. 10). Palmer calls on us to listen, and to let our being—our vocation—speak. To Palmer, this inner being is our authentic path in the world;

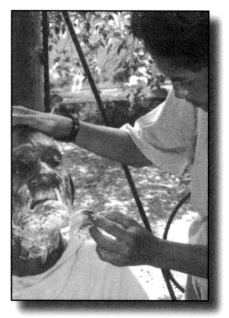

to live the life that wants to live within us is to live authentically, to be our authentic selves.

Christiansen (1999), on the other hand, presented a different view of the self and our inner being. According to Christiansen, goals help define our selves in that they generate images of our *possible selves* (Markus & Nurius, 1986). Goals are viewed in the context of the self: "Goals that individuals view as important, and to which they are committed, are effective because these goals are self-relevant and self-defining" (Christiansen, p. 553). Christiansen proposed that, since occupation is goal-directed activity, occupation, too, exists within the context of the self. Goal-directed activity and the self are bound to each other. To Christiansen, selfhood presents itself in our lives in the form of goals and occupation; setting goals and engaging in occupation constitute important dimensions of our being in this world.

Surely the man in the nursing home who was enabled by the therapist to whittle and carve was once again living with day-to-day goals ("we had him looking forward to getting up in the morning") and opportunities to engage in occupation within the context of his self. Viewed from Christiansen's (1999) perspective, whittling and carving were self-relevant and self-defining occupations for him. Through the use of occupation, the gentleman again "knew" his self and he was able to express his inner self to his immediate world. But we can also interpret the happenings in the therapist's story by using Palmer's (2000) concept of authentic selfhood. We could say that the therapist, with her sensitive approach to getting to know the man, successfully created possibilities for him to live his authentic self. The move to a nursing home—with the potential abrupt loss of all familiar routines, surroundings, and daily occupations—is clearly an event that can prevent a person from living authentically. Real life and the real self may no longer be present in the world of an institution, unless enabled to be there. At least to some extent, the therapist could be said to have enabled the man to live the life that was within him. And he became a happy man.

## *Being and Occupational Therapy*

Palmer (2000) and Christiansen (1999) offer us ways to think about our being in this world. The story of the occupational therapist and the man in the nursing home is a story of one older person's way of being in the world as transformed by the occupations of whittling and carving. The following narrative about a therapist's experience of working with an 8-month-old baby boy serves to illustrate that these concepts of *being* and occupational therapy are applicable across the life span.

> The case was an 8-month-old boy who had a spinal cord injury at T2-3 sustained in an automobile accident. The baby was very social, smiling and babbling in response to holding and talking. He enjoyed batting at toys in a side lying position, but he could not sit up for play. Because of the paralysis, sitting him up in a high chair for feeding or play was not possible. After therapy sessions, he would cry when placed back in bed, even if he was propped in side lying with toys in view. His crying was not angry or frustrated, simply sad and continuous until he was picked up or fell asleep.

We determined that he was happy in a supported sitting position, not semi-reclined in an infant seat. In this position, he would play by himself, knocking toys around on a tray, or watching the nursing staff.

I designed a supportive vest using Ace bandage wrap to support his abdominal muscles for breathing and Velcro so that he could sit in a high chair. The first day he had it, he smiled and laughed for the whole time I was with him. … He ate his lunch for the first time in a sitting position, and cried when his nurse tried to put him to bed. She decided to leave him in the chair for another 5 minutes, and he fell asleep in his support in the high chair.

Nursing staff loved the support because he was so much more independent. His mom liked it because he looked more "normal." And he loved it; he cried consistently when we took him out of it. I felt very "OT-ish." (Hasselkus & Dickie, 1994)

Even an 8-month-old baby has an authentic self, for as Palmer (2000) stated, we are born with a life to be lived. To me, this story is about a therapist who enabled the baby to live more authentically. The therapist changed one aspect of the baby's way of being in the world back to what his authentic way had been before the car accident—sitting in a high chair, playing with toys and eating, being able to interact with his environment. In the supportive vest, the baby was able to express his selfhood through occupation and, we might say, was able to get to know his self through occupation. He was, once again, able to let his life speak.

But there is more in this story than the baby's selfhood and recovered ability to let his life speak. Also present is the selfhood of the occupational therapist. At the end of her story, the therapist says, "I felt very OT-ish." What a wonderful statement of authentic being! From her experience with the baby came a sense that *her* life was speaking. In Palmer's words, she was living the life she was meant to live; she was doing what she was meant to do. From Christiansen's perspective, the possible selves that the occupational therapist imagined for both the baby and herself—her imagined ways of being in the world—had been realized. The therapist had used occupation to bring this about: thinking about the baby's capabilities; identifying his times of happiness; problem-solving how to maximize the baby's capabilities and happiness; designing a supportive vest and trying it out; watching for the responses of the baby, the nurses, and the mother; judging the success of the vest by the baby's way of being—"And he loved it,"—and what the vest seemed to mean to the others in the story.

Isn't this what occupational therapy is all about? Might we not think of our work as directed toward enabling people, as best as possible, to live the lives that lie within them? Whatever their ages, whatever their capabilities and disabilities, whatever their circumstances—we are, in effect, working together with our clients to let their lives speak, to enable the expression of their authentic selves, to help them experience their own deep inner beings in their daily lives. And we do this through occupation. At the same time, we are working with our clients to let our *own* lives speak. Not only do we seek to understand and enter the lives of those with whom we work, not only do we seek to create together a treatment process that becomes a story with meaningfulness to us and to our clients (Mattingly & Fleming, 1994), but we also seek to let *our* lives speak through this treatment process (Hasselkus & Dickie, 1994; Rosa & Hasselkus, 1996). For those of us who are occupational therapists, to feel "very OT-ish" is to feel very authentic. As it is for all human beings, our daily occupation potentially contributes to our authentic way of being in the world.

# OCCUPATION AND BECOMING

*Becoming* is a term that "holds the notions of potential and growth, of transformation and self-actualization" (Wilcock, 1998a, p. 251). Wilcock believed that, as occupational therapists, we are part of our clients' *becomings*—that is, we share in the potential and growth that is experienced by the people with whom we work. In her view, people "need to be enabled towards what they are best fitted, and wishful to become" (p. 251); occupational therapists act as such enablers. This view, that we are needed to proactively take part in the creation of others' life stories in order to actualize the potential that lies within them, is a view that incorporates both Christensen's (1999) and Palmer's (2000) views on being and becoming. As I stated above, according to Christiansen, goals help generate images of our possible selves; goals that individuals view as important are self-relevant and self-defining (Christiansen). At the same time, one's *potential* is that which lies within, waiting to unfold, so to speak. Christiansen is for helping the unfolding process through occupation and therapy; Palmer's approach is more one of watching and listening to see what unfolds—not getting in the way of the unfolding, but also not taking proactive action to assist in the process that is taking place.

## The Therapist–Client Interaction as It Unfolds

To live the life that lies within us or to proactively create the life for which we have potential—these are two views of *becoming* proposed by Palmer (2000) and Christiansen (1999), respectively.

These theoretical frameworks of lifespan development are instructive to our thinking about occupation therapy and *becoming*. First, we can think of the changes that the therapist seeks to bring about in a client during therapy as one aspect of a person's "development." As therapy takes place, the nature of the interaction between the therapist and the client may reflect a succession of theoretical approaches. If the therapist approaches the interaction from a model of therapist-as-expert, the therapist–client relationship will reflect beliefs that the influence of the therapist (the environment) is absolutely necessary in order for change or development to occur (we need to help bring about the client's full potential). If the therapist approaches the interaction from a model of therapist-as-partner, the relationship may reflect a more dialectic theory of becoming, with therapist and client contributing more equally to the process of change that is brought about during the therapy. Finally, if the therapist approaches the interaction from a client-centered perspective, then the outcomes of therapy will represent more of an unfolding process, with the change evolving strongly from the client's inner potential. All of these approaches represent ways for the therapist to use occupation to enable the becoming of a client.

In point of fact, therapists are likely to use more than one theoretical framework as they carry out therapy with clients; shifting from the therapist-as-expert to the partnership and, finally, to the client-centered approach to therapy may reflect a natural developmental sequence in therapeutic relationships. We may start out with a client by using a fairly directive approach in our therapy. As therapy progresses and the client becomes more engaged, we gradually shift to a partnership approach with joint planning and sharing in the therapy process. Ideally, we may reach a point in the therapeutic relationship in which the client is the dominant figure, making the major decisions and acting more autonomously in the therapy process as ultimate independence from therapy draws near.

## *Occupation on the Rocks: A Clinical Example of Becoming*

We derive satisfaction from our work when we believe we have had some kind of impact on another person's way of being in the world (Hasselkus & Dickie, 1994). We strive to set measurable short- and long-term goals to be able to describe the changes that have occurred as the therapy has progressed. In carrying out the therapeutic process, we believe that we are facilitating the *becoming* of the people with whom we work. In the therapy story below, all three approaches to therapy may be discerned—therapist as expert, therapist and patient in partnership, and client-centered therapy.

> The setting was a craft clinic where individual patients were sent by prescription by ward psychiatrists or psychologists. ... I utilized the lapidary for many patients who had trouble identifying with arts and crafts as a masculine activity.

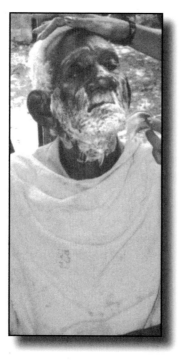

> I remember one patient in particular who stated that he was not interested in "this kindergarten stuff" upon his first visit to the clinic where he saw a lot of table crafts in process. From his therapy order and my interview with him, I found out he was a tree trimmer and was used to heavy outdoor work. I introduced him to my "rock pile" and he became intrigued by the slabbing machine that cut rocks into slices to be worked into stones to set into jewelry findings. He stated he always wanted to see what was inside some of the rocks he picked up in the forest, and later he did bring in some of his own rocks.

> He was in the hospital as an alternative to jail due to the fact he had broken a restraining order to keep away from his ex-wife. He was very bitter about his marriage break-up and not being able to see his children.

Once he learned how to use the saw, he continued to slab rocks daily for several weeks, maintaining a good supply for the clinic. I introduced him to my volunteer who took care of the lapidary equipment for me, and who also had become quite skilled at all aspects of lapidary and jewelry making. The two worked together well and taught other patients these skills as well. Before this patient left the hospital he had bought equipment to continue this craft and a station wagon to transport it all back to his home state. By this time, he had become much calmer and able to discuss the deterioration of the marriage, his feelings about it, and to start to plan for his future. He wrote to me periodically over the next few years and the last time I heard from him, he was going to be married. …

I felt good about his progress and the unit staff gave me much credit for helping him turn his life around. After this episode, I used this craft successfully many times. (Hasselkus & Dickie)

In this narrative about a satisfying experience in practice, an occupational therapist describes her interactions with a client in a psychiatric craft clinic in a way that clearly reveals three philosophies of human development. Initially, she is directive (she speaks of his therapy "order" and states "I introduced him to my rock pile"), reflecting her belief that it is up to her to make something happen here. Her initial direction of the client to the lapidary area is followed by the gradual beginnings of sharing—first, shared interests ("he stated he always wanted to see what was inside some of the rocks he picked up in the forest") and later sharing work and responsibilities ("I introduced him to my volunteer. … The two worked together well and taught other patients these skills as well"). Finally, "Before this patient left the hospital, he had bought equipment to continue this craft and a station wagon to transport it all back to his home"; these were actions that reflected autonomous decision making as the therapy and hospitalization drew to an end.

Through the therapy process, the client's *becoming* has been facilitated. The therapist who related the narrative described what she had done with the client as "helping him turn his life around." She actually used the word "become," stating that, "By this time, he had become much calmer and able to discuss the deterioration of the marriage. …" This man was also now able to "start to plan for his future"; in other words, the client was able once again to take part in his own becoming, his own continuing development as he lived into his own future.

Just as we saw hints of the therapist's being in the earlier narrative about the 8-month-old baby, in this narrative we find hints about the therapist's becoming, expressed in her words, "After this episode, I used this craft successfully many times." This lapidary "episode" changed the therapist as well as the client. New understandings of lapidary as a meaningful occupation and its potential contribution to the being and becoming of clients led to the therapist's use of the craft many more times. Even though crafts may no longer be the primary modality of occupational therapy in psychosocial care, the same process of becoming accompanies practice today with whatever modalities are being used. Our own occupation also contributes to our own becoming; "doing" occupational therapy is one way that we accomplish "selfing," that we let our lives speak, and that we become.

# OCCUPATION AND BELONGING

"Homeless Man Dies on Capitol Bench." This was the headline for a small front page article in my hometown daily newspaper one day in June 2009 (Bargnes, 2009). Not until the next day was his identity determined; by the day after that, officials were "still attempting to contact" his family. A downtown worker who had tried to befriend the man was quoted as saying, "He clearly lacked the mental ability to live by himself … he was a very kind and gentle man; he slipped through the cracks."

The sense of aloneness in this "homeless" man's life is profound. Upon reading the article, I was immediately struck by the isolation of this human being in the midst (literally) of a vibrant Midwestern city. Recent research data and theory-building (Hammell, 2009a; Rebeiro et al., 2001; Wilcock, 2006) have proposed that "belonging" is a basic human need—crucial to well-being and survival. According to Rebeiro et al., belonging needs include the need for a place that is physically and emotionally safe, provides both private and community spaces, meets social needs, and helps to form a group identity (p. 497). It seems that "Dwayne," the homeless man who died on the capitol bench, had no such place in his life; this was a man who "lingered on a heating grate" near an office building in winter and who spent "little if any time at a shelter" (Bargnes, 2009). His everyday life was one of *not* belonging.

Dwayne's life situation helps illustrate the reasons for occupational therapy to expand beyond its traditional focus on individuals to focus also on social systems, communities, and populations. In other words, in addition to our deep and appropriate concern for individuals such as Dwayne, we need also to focus our attention on the social and community systems to bring about changes that might offer more effective assistance and better meet the needs of people with these vulnerabilities—including the need to "belong." How and why did Dwayne "slip through the cracks?" What services and resources might have enabled this "kind and gentle man" to live and die in a more humane and less solitary way? How can occupation-based programming contribute to a better quality of life for at-risk populations in our world—helping them to meet their needs of being, becoming and belonging?

## Occupational Injustice

A concept developing in recent years is that of *occupational injustice* (Townsend & Wilcock, 2004; Whiteford, 2003). Occupational injustices include phenomena such as prolonged experiences of disconnectedness and isolation, limited choices in occupation due to disability and stereotyping, exclusion from mainstream life, and lack of opportunity for everyday choices and decision making (Townsend & Wilcock). A homeless person such as Dwayne was likely experiencing many aspects of occupational injustice. Surely a man who spent his days in winter "lingering on a heating grate" and who slept and died on a public bench on the grounds of the state capitol was living his days with very few choices and long periods of disconnectedness.

Many aspects of occupational injustice act as barriers to people's needs for "belonging." Townsend and Wilcock urged occupational therapy practitioners and researchers to engage in "critical analysis of the everyday lives of our populations of concern, the systems in which we work, and our profession" (2004, p. 84). Populations that would benefit from such an approach are people who live in poverty, experience violence on a day-to-day basis, perform demeaning work with low wages, live in refugee confinement or prison systems, are homeless, and are dependent on systems that discriminate on the basis of disability as related to housing, health care, education, and transportation. Ruth Watson (2004) succinctly summarized the therapist's role in addressing such social concerns as that of providing a "situational diagnosis, informed by the power structures that operate within the chosen circumstances" (p. 61). The most difficult aspect of the therapist's role in arriving at this situational diagnosis is the question of how to negotiate, define, and maintain boundaries (p. 62).

## Dignity in the Dining Room

The following narrative from an occupational therapist in a long-term-care facility for older people in the United States provides testimony to the difficulties and fragility present in such situations. The issues of power, boundaries, and complexity are clearly illustrated.

> [In the nursing home] there were quite a few folks who were not feeding themselves for one reason or another, and I saw a great need for these folks, if they were able to feed themselves, to go ahead and do that. There were a lot of people who were aware and didn't want the food stuffed down them and wanted to take their time eating. The lack of dignity that happened when they weren't able to feed themselves was really showing.

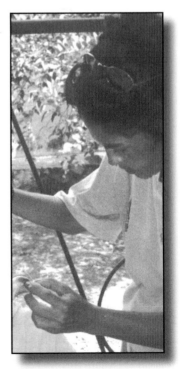

> So I gave a feeding in-service, and I wrote this all up and I recommended that they go ahead and let some of these people feed themselves and not separate—there was a "feeders" room and a regular dining room—and just try to integrate them. And if some of the other people needed help, then some of the more able-bodied maybe could help, and so there would be just more of a sense of community there.

> So I wrote that up to that effect. The director of nursing was all for it, [but] the administrator called me in and said, "I want this rewritten," because one of the things they needed to do was, after we gave our reports, they needed then to follow through to get their accreditation. And I said, "You know, I can't re-write this. I can't ethically do that because I see this as a real need, and I don't see this as optional." And, oh, he went on to tell me

that he would have my job and that I would never come back. There were other incidents like that where I would recommend a specific activity or treatment and he would buck that, and I ended up voluntarily not working in that system anymore ... I mean, he was too powerful. I had real mixed feelings about [leaving]—on the one hand, I was on the side of the fence that I will do this until I see some changes, but on the other hand, it was a corporate nursing home and it was just bigger than life, basically. Bigger than me, that's for sure.

This therapist did her best to make a "situational diagnosis" about the current practices of her facility, with the hope of bringing about an improved quality of life and a reduced level of occupational injustice for the residents. In the terminology of occupational injustice, the residents who were being fed in this nursing home were experiencing exclusion from mainstream life in the facility (the "regular" dining room), a form of demeaning occupational segregation based on disability (relegated to the "feeders'" room), social exclusion and restriction of social opportunities, and subjection to a system that prioritized efficiencies in time and place over resident choice and decision making—all due to factors outside of the residents' control.

The occupational therapist's goal was to create, instead, an eating experience that would lead to a feeling of community and relationship—in other words, a sense of group identity and belonging instead of occupational marginalization, deprivation, and alienation. This therapist wisely had sought support for her proposal from the head nurse, but the administrator seemed to be adamantly opposed to her ideas. Boundaries for policy making and change clearly needed to be defined and negotiated in this situation.

Perhaps inclusion of the administrator in the initial exploration and development of the proposal would have led to a different outcome. Or, perhaps not. Issues addressed at the system or population level require "the integration and thoughtful reconstruction of a large amount of information to arrive at a situational diagnosis" (Watson, 2004, p. 61). As Townsend and Wilcock stated, we need to develop "critical, reflexive rather than technical, prescriptive practice" (2004, p. 84). With her proposal for a different dining program, the therapist at the nursing home was demonstrating critical, reflexive thinking and ideas at the system level. She was striving to address the existing policies of the facility, policies that flew in the face of community and belonging and led to occupational injustices. But trying to sort out and understand the layers upon layers of power and decision-making entities (head nurse, administrator, accreditation agency, etc.)—present in some form in all occupational settings—can be overwhelming and defeating. As we venture further into this new professional emphasis on effecting occupational changes within groups, systems, and populations, we will need curriculum and training modifications to help us develop the skills needed to be effective in these domains.

To repeat the quotation from Crabtree (1998) used at the beginning of the chapter, "The nature of humans is to make meaning through occupation." For ourselves and for the people with whom we work, occupation contributes to our being, our becoming, and our belonging. With occupation as the core concept of our profession, we are, by default, custodians of meaning and meaning-givers.

# REFERENCES

American Occupational Therapy Association. (1993). Position paper: Purposeful activity. *American Journal of Occupational Therapy, 47*, 1081-1082.

American Occupational Therapy Association. (1995). Position paper: Occupation. *American Journal of Occupational Therapy, 49*, 1015-1018.

American Occupational Therapy Association (2008). Occupational therapy practice framework: Domain & process (2nd ed.). *American Journal of Occupational Therapy, 62*, 625-683.

Bargnes, K. (2009, June 17). Homeless man dies on capitol bench. *Wisconsin State Journal.*

Blakeney, A. B., & Marshall, A. (2009). Water quality, health, and human occupations. *American Journal of Occupational Therapy, 63*, 46-57.

Bonder, B. R. (2006). Family occupations in later life. *Journal of Occupational Science, 13*, 107-116.

Braveman, B., & Bass-Haugen, J. (2009). Editorial: Social justice and health disparities: An evolving discourse in occupational therapy research and intervention. *American Journal of Occupational Therapy, 63*, 7-12.

Canadian Association of Occupational Therapy. (1997). *Enabling occupation: An occupational therapy perspective.* Ottawa, Ontario, Canada: CAOT Publishers, ACE.

Canadian Association of Occupational Therapy. (2002). *Enabling occupation: An occupational therapy perspective* (3rd ed.). Ottawa, Ontario, Canada: CAOT Publishers, ACE.

Christiansen, C. (1999). Defining lives: Occupation as identity: An essay on competence, coherence, and the creation of meaning. *American Journal of Occupational Therapy, 53*, 547-558.

Clark, F., Parham, D., Carlson, M., Frank, G., Jackson, J., Pierce, D., ... Zemke, R. (1991). Occupational science: Academic innovation in the service of occupational therapy's future. *American Journal of Occupational Therapy, 45*, 300-310.

Crabtree, J. L. (1998). The end of occupational therapy. *American Journal of Occupational Therapy, 52*, 205-214.

DeGrace, B. W. (2003). Occupation-based and family-centered care: A challenge for current practice. *American Journal of Occupational Therapy, 57*, 347-350.

DeGroat, E. J., Lyons, K. D., & Tickle-Degnen, L. (2006). Favorite activity interview as a window into the identity of people with Parkinson's disease. *OTJR: Occupation, Participation and Health, 26*, 56-68.

Dickie, V. (2009). What is occupation? In E. B. Crepeau, E. S. Cohn, & B. A. Boyt Schell (Eds.), *Willard & Spackman's occupational therapy* (11th ed., pp. 15-21). Philadelphia, PA: Lippincott Williams & Wilkins.

Dickie, V., Cutchin, M. P., & Humphry, R. (2006). Occupation as transactional experience; A critique of individualism in occupational science. *Journal of Occupational Science, 13*, 83-93.

Engelhardt, T. (1983). Occupational therapists as technologists and custodians of meaning. In G. Kielhofner (Ed.), *Health through occupation* (pp. 139-144). Philadelphia, PA: F. A. Davis.

Golledge, J. (1998). Distinguishing between occupation, purposeful activity and activity, Part 1: Review and explanation. *British Journal of Occupational Therapy, 61*, 99-105.

Hammell, K. W. (2004). Dimensions of meaning in the occupations of daily life. *Canadian Journal of Occupational Therapy, 71*, 296-305.

Hammell, K. W. (2008). Reflections on well-being and occupational rights. *Canadian Journal of Occupational Therapy, 75*, 61-64.

Hammell, K. W. (2009a). Sacred texts: A skeptical exploration of the assumptions underpinning theories of occupation. *Canadian Journal of Occupational Therapy, 76*, 6-13.

Hammell, K. W. (2009b). Self-care, productivity, and leisure, or dimensions of occupational experience? Rethinking occupational categories. *Canadian Journal of Occupational Therapy, 76,* 107-114.

Hasselkus, B. R. (2006). Eleanor Clarke Slagle Lecture. The world of everyday occupation: Real people, real lives. *American Journal of Occupational Therapy, 60,* 627-640.

Hasselkus, B. R., & Dickie, V. A. (1994). Doing occupational therapy: Dimensions of satisfaction and dissatisfaction. *American Journal of Occupational Therapy, 48,* 145-154.

Iwama, M. (2005). Situated meaning: An issue of culture, inclusion, and occupational therapy. In F. Kronenberg, S. S. Algado, & N. Pollard (Eds.), *Occupational therapy without borders* (pp. 127-139). Edinburgh, UK: Churchill Livingstone Elsevier.

Jonsson, H. (2008). A new direction in the conceptualization and categorization of occupation. *Journal of Occupational Science, 15,* 3-8.

Kegan, R. (1982). *The evolving self.* Cambridge, MA: Harvard University Press.

Kronenberg, F., Algado, A. A., & Pollard, N. (2005). *Occupational therapy without borders: Learning the spirit of survivors.* London, UK: Elsevier.

Law, M., Polatajko, H., Baptiste, S., & Townsend, E. (1997). Core concepts of occupational therapy. In E. Townsend (Ed.), *Enabling occupation: An occupational therapy perspective* (pp. 29-56). Ottawa, ON: CAOT Publishers, ACE.

Markus, H., & Nurius, P. S. (1986). Possible selves. *American Psychology, 41,* 954-969.

Mattingly, C., & Fleming, M. (1994). Interactive reasoning: Collaborating with the person. In C. Mattingly & M. H. Fleming (Eds.), *Clinical reasoning: Forms of inquiry in a therapeutic practice* (pp. 178-196). Philadelphia, PA: F. A. Davis.

McAdams, D. P. (1997). The case for unity in (post) modern self. In R. D. Ashmore & L. Jussim (Eds.), *Self and identity: Fundamental issues* (pp. 46-78). New York, NY: Oxford University Press.

Nelson, D. L. (1996). Therapeutic occupation: A definition. *American Journal of Occupational Therapy, 50,* 775-782.

Palmer, P. J. (2000). *Let your life speak: Listening for the voice of vocation.* San Francisco, CA: Jossey-Bass.

Parham, D. (1998). What is the proper domain of occupational therapy research? *American Journal of Occupational Therapy, 52,* 485-489.

Pierce, D. (2001). Untangling occupation and activity. *American Journal of Occupational Therapy, 55,* 138-146.

Primeau, L. A. (1998). Orchestration of work and play within families. *American Journal of Occupational Therapy, 52,* 188-195.

Rebeiro, K. L., Day, D., Semeniuk, B., O'Brien, M., & Wilson, B. (2001). Northern initiative for social action: An occupation-based mental health program. *American Journal of Occupational Therapy, 55,* 493-500.

Rosa, S., & Hasselkus, B. R. (1996). Connecting with patients: The personal experience of professional helping. *Occupational Therapy Journal of Research, 16,* 245-260.

Townsend, E., & Wilcock, A. A. (2004). Occupational justice and client-centered practice: A dialogue in progress. *Canadian Journal of Occupational Therapy, 71,* 75-87.

Trombly, C. A. (1995). Occupation, purposefulness and meaningfulness as therapeutic mechanisms. *American Journal of Occupational Therapy, 49,* 960-972.

Watson, R. (2004). A population approach to transformation. In R. Watson & L. Swartz (Eds.), *Transformation through occupation* (pp. 51-65). London, UK: Whurr Pub.

Watson, R., & Fourie, M. (2004). International and African influences on occupational therapy. In R. Watson & L. Swartz (Eds.), *Transformation through occupation* (pp. 33-50). London, UK: Whurr Pub.

Watson, R., & Swartz, L. (Eds.) (2004). *Transformation through occupation*. London,UK: Whurr Pub.

Whiteford, G. (2003). When people cannot participate: Occupational deprivation. In C. Christiansen & E. Townsend (Eds.), *An introduction to occupation: The art and science of living* (pp. 221-242). Upper Saddle River, NJ: Prentice Hall.

Wilcock, A. A. (1998a). *An occupational perspective of health*. Thorofare, NJ: SLACK Incorporated.

Wilcock, A. A. (1998b). Reflections on doing, being and becoming. *Canadian Journal of Occupational Therapy, 65,* 248-256.

Wilcock, A. A. (2006). *An occupational perspective of health* (2nd ed.). Thorofare, NJ: SLACK Incorporated.

Yerxa, E. (1994). Dreams, dilemmas, and decisions for occupational therapy practice in a new millenium: An American perspective. *American Journal of Occupational Therapy, 48,* 586-589.

Zemke, R., & Clark, F. (1996). *Occupational science: An evolving discipline*. Philadelphia, PA: F. A. Davis.

# C H A P T E R   3

# SPACE AND PLACE: SOURCES OF MEANING IN OCCUPATION

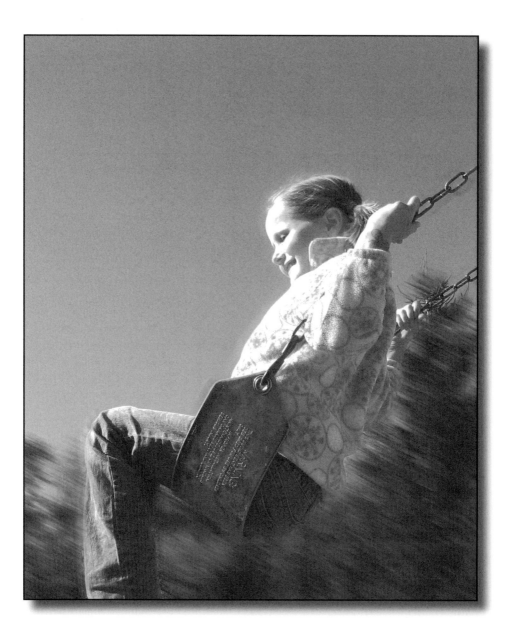

How do you like to go up in a swing,
Up in the air so blue?
Oh, I do think it the pleasantest thing
Ever a child can do!

From "The Swing," by Robert Louis Stevenson (n.d.)

I grew up having a swing in the backyard. The swing hung by two ropes from a strong branch on a bur oak, and the seat was a wooden board with a hole drilled in each end through which the rope was tied. The swing was, actually, the only piece of play equipment we had in our yard. Perhaps because of that, my sister and I and our friends played hard on that swing, devoting much play time to "pushing" each other, trying to pump high enough to touch a tree branch with our feet, twisting the rope up as tight as we could and then climbing on the seat and spinning free, taking turns to pump up higher and higher and then leaping off the swing to try to beat the record for leaping the farthest, and playing a game called "circus" in which we made up "tricks" to do on the swing, imagining ourselves as performers on a trapeze.

I have a powerful sense of "place" connected with that childhood swing. The swing itself, the tree, the patch of bare ground under the swing where the grass never grew, and the grassy lawn around the swing constitute a place of meaning for me. Vivid memories of my childhood swing as place have come back to me recently, jogged by my preparations for writing this chapter.

The geographer Tuan (1977) has said, "Place is an organized world of meaning. It is essentially a static concept. If we see the world as process, constantly changing, we should not be able to develop any sense of place" (p. 179). A sense of place "holds." My memories of the swing have form and structure and contain certain things—they are an organized world of meaning. The swing, as place, holds; it remains the same as always (de Certeau, 1984; Tuan).

In this chapter, we will think about the meaning of place and space in our lives and their relationships to everyday occupation and to occupational therapy. The concept of *placelessness* is introduced. Particular attention is paid to home as a space and place and to the meaning of *homeyness*. The special places of our lives are explored, including the places of childhood. Finally, understandings of a geography of health and well-being within space and place are put forward.

## SPACE AND PLACE IN OUR LIVES

We often think of place as a designation for a location or site, but it is much more than that; in fact, Langer (1953) has argued that location is merely an incidental quality of place. In addition to the setting, a sense of place may include "landscape, ritual, routine, other people, personal experiences, care and concern for home" and the context of other places (Relph, 1976, p. 29). The key aspect in this listing of ingredients is personal experience. Casey (1987) called place a "container of experiences" (p. 186). It might be more accurate to say that place is a container of *memories* of experiences. Stegner (1992) has said, "A place is not a place until people have been born in it, have grown up in it, lived in it, known it, died in it—have both experienced and shaped it, as individuals, families, neighborhoods, and communities. ... No place is a place until things that have happened in it are remembered" (pp. 201-202).

Casey (1987) referred to this phenomenological link between remembering and place as "place memory" (p. 181). Place memory is not limited to remembered time, although such temporal aspects of memory have been the focus of most memory

Hasselkus, B. R.
*The Meaning of Everyday Occupation, Second Edition* (pp. 41-60).

research (the terms *short-term memory* and *long-term memory* come quickly to mind). Place memory is memory of *"having been in a place"* (Casey, p. 183). My memories of the swing are place memories; they are intimate memories of my *lived* experiences on the swing.

Place is a part of *space*, but at the same time place is set apart from space by the intentions and concentrated attention that it harbors. My childhood swing is a part of the backyard space, but at the same time it is set apart from the rest of the yard space by virtue of the fact that it was the focus of so much attention and activity and because of the experiences with other people, the routines of play, and the landscape of home with which it is associated.

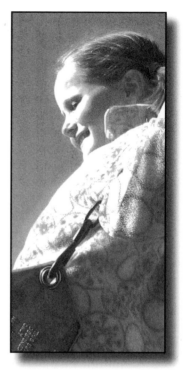

Space, then, is often conceptualized as a larger, more abstract, and more neutral entity than place. Casey (1996) described *space* as a "neutral, pre-given medium, a tabula rasa onto which the particularities of culture and history come to be inscribed, with place as the presumed result" (p. 14). Space *is*. As human beings, we live in the context of a basic spatiality that is unselfconsciously structured by our own experiences. From infancy onward, as we move about in our worlds and respond sensorially to the world, we become spatially attuned, understanding the dimensions of up and down, left and right, in front of and behind, within sight and beyond sight, within reach and beyond reach (Relph, 1976). As we build experience into our lives, we create places out of spaces, or as Tuan put it, "What begins as undifferentiated space becomes place as we get to know it better and endow it with value" (1977, p. 6).

## HEALTH AND WELL-BEING WITHIN SPACE AND PLACE

The relationship between space and place and health is complicated. On the one hand, we have the rather subtle sense of well-being and comfort that we experience when we feel that a place is "right" in terms of its size, design, décor, colors, location, source of light, temperature, etc. This sense of well-being is one kind of "being in place" (Rowles, 1991, 2000, 2008); that is, a way to be at one with one's lifeworld. In some situations, certain aspects of an environment are believed to promote actual recovery and healing after trauma or illness, as well as to support general well-being (Leibrock, 2000; Tyson, 1998). Cutchin (2005) used the term *therapeutic landscapes* to refer to the healing effects of places with special meaningfulness.

The ancient Chinese art of *feng shui* offers another way to express the sense of harmony one can feel within an environment. Good *feng shui* means that a place has good chemistry for us, it suits us, and we really like being in the place (Woon, 1991). On the other hand, according to the art of *feng shui*, many characteristics of the environment can work to a person's *dis*advantage, such as having a road or sharp edge of a building located in such a way that it points directly at you when you look out the window of your office or home.

A strong feeling that one is in the "wrong" place can have deleterious effects on health; anyone who has experienced homesickness understands the misery of such a feeling only too well. And what feels right for one person may feel wrong for another, as becomes all too obvious when traveling with a companion and trying to agree on a bed and breakfast place to stay the night.

What occurs in the interaction between place and person in everyday life can have both subtle and dramatic, positive and negative effects on people's sense of well-being and health (Kearns, 1993). These considerations and examples fit into the larger occupational framework of the person–environment or person–context transactional models of occupational therapy (Dickie, Cutchin, & Humphry, 2006; Dunn, Brown, & McGuigan, 1994; Law et al., 1996; Pierce, Munier, & Myers, 2009). The basic premise of these models is the belief that occupational performance results from the dynamic relationship between people and the environments in which they carry out their everyday lives. Pushing the model of transactionalism further, Dickie et al. voiced their discomfort with the dualism of person–environment models. They call for "a transactional occupational science based on Dewey" (p. 91), one that conceptualizes the transactional unit (person and environment) as a whole (i.e., as co-constitutive). Each must be seen as part of the other, and "occupation can be viewed as a transaction joining person and situation" (p. 90). Space and place are aspects of this transactional unit, helping to constitute the meaning and choices of occupation in which people engage. All these factors *together* influence people's health and well-being.

## SPACE AND THERAPY

In occupational therapy, we at times focus on the elemental movement of the body in space. We assess the ability of a client to move his or her body in space, to transfer from one stable surface to another, to ambulate through space, to turn in space, to bend and twist in space without loss of balance, to carry objects in space, to use assistive devices such as walkers or canes or wheelchairs or wheeled carts to move about in space, to reach objects that are needed within a space, to be able to go into and out of spaces. For some clients, we may direct our attention to the perceptual components of spatiality, assessing their spatial perception abilities such as depth, height, directionality, verticality, and rotation. If, in our assessment, we find that a client's abilities are impaired in any of these areas, then we carry out therapeutic treatments to enable them to regain or attain abilities in these body skills so they may move about in their life spaces and interact with their environments as best as possible.

In addition to the body and its personal space, occupational therapists assess external spaces such as workspaces and spaces within the home, school, and community (Pohl et al., 2006; Sanford, Pynoos, Tejral, & Browne, 2002). We evaluate architectural and ergonomic factors so that barriers to body movement within these spaces may be eliminated and effective movement may be enhanced. Accessibility within space is emphasized—that is, a person's ability to safely negotiate movement in and throughout the necessary and desired spaces of the everyday world around us. As therapists, we modify the spaces in people's lives—adding grab bars, railings, electronic devices, ramps; widening doorways; removing sills; lowering work surfaces—to maximize safe mobility and usability (Erikson, Karlsson, Söderström, & Tham, 2005; Fänge & Iwarsson, 2005).

Architect David Seamon (2002) has reminded us of the reciprocal relationship between social life and the built environment and the importance of habitual movement in our home spaces in our everyday lives. In work related to space and occupational therapy, researchers at the Center on Everyday Lives of Families (CELF) in Los Angeles are studying houses as a part of family culture and focusing on the compatibility of housing designs with the activity needs and patterns of families (Graesch, 2004). The CELF research seeks to address questions about how "modern-day Los Angeles families use their house spaces" to interact, do chores, and to carry out job- and school-related work in their daily lives (p. 20). Research such as this can help occupational therapists better effect home modifications responsive to specific family needs and everyday experiences. As occupational therapy personnel, we can see and utilize the connections between Seamon's concept of habitual movement in the home and Graesch's findings that 73% of everyday family activities take place in the kitchen and family room. The two sisters in the narrative below refused to consider the therapist's initial recommendations for home adaptations, placing a higher priority on being able to maintain their usual habitual patterns of movement and activity in their home than on making changes that would ease the demands of their caregiving situation.

In order for *place* to be a part of our therapy, we need to consider the *meaning* of space as well as clients' spatial perceptual skills and the accessibility features of their environments. Once meaning is brought into the picture, we have shifted our attention from space to place.

# FROM SPACE TO PLACE IN THERAPY

Gitlin, Corcoran, and Leinmiller-Eckhardt (1995) provided a compelling example of the difference between space and place in the lives of clients. They told the story of an occupational therapist in home care and her first visit to the home of two sisters who were caring for one sister's 89-year-old husband who had dementia. Impressed with the enormous difficulty imposed on the two elderly sisters as they cared for a resistive man twice their size, the occupational therapist made the following recommendations: (a) the use of formal home care services; (b) major home modifications such as a stair glide or moving the husband's bed downstairs; (c) medical intervention for the husband's poor nutritional status; and (d) day care participation and preparation for possible nursing home placement for the husband. The sisters rejected all of these recommendations.

As she thought more about the situation, the occupational therapist slowly realized that her recommendations reflected only her own perspective, one that focused on the medical and dysfunctional aspects of the situation. With continued observation and careful listening, the therapist came to understand that the "essential meaning of the caregiving activities for these two frail women was to maintain a sense of normalcy with the way things were before the onset of [the husband's] dementia" (Gitlin et al., 1995, p. 806). Normalcy meant maintaining the husband's daily routines of eating, resting, and moving about the house (habitual movement patterns) as they had been throughout his adult life, imposing minimal changes on what he used to do and how he used to be. Working within the framework of these new understandings of the meaning of the situation to the family caregivers, the occupational therapist was able to offer a number of solutions that both eased the stresses of the caregivers' tasks as well as upheld the biographical image of the husband.

All people face challenges of changing circumstances throughout their lives—challenges that often require us to reshape our home and community spaces. Cutchin (2003) has coined the term *place integration* to designate this reshaping process, applying the concept to what others have called the phenomenon of aging-in-place. In the case example above, the occupational therapist first approached the people in their home as people within a space; the space was seen as "neutral," without special meanings, and recommendations for changes in the space and routines within the space were formulated based on the therapist's perceptions of the risk and impairment that was present. But these recommendations were rejected. The house was not simply neutral space to the three people in this family; the house was, instead, "an organized world of meaning"—a place. Once the therapist recognized the "placeness" of the home, she was able to begin to connect with these clients and work together with them to develop acceptable solutions to their problems—to help them through the process of place integration.

What this story means to me is this: As therapists, we come into people's lives at some point in their already ongoing life narratives (Helfrich, Kielhofner, & Mattingly, 1994; Mattingly, 1994). When we are in their lifeworlds—their homes, schools, work settings—we are in locations that have experiential memories attached to them. We are in *places* with people who have place memories. Our task is to come to understand the meaning of those places and then to fit into those meanings as best as we can. Otherwise, our treatment goals and recommendations are likely to be rejected, as assuredly as were those of the occupational therapist in the case study.

## PLACELESSNESS

*Placelessness* is a word used by Relph (1976) and means the absence of experience of place except at the superficial and casual level. A lack of awareness of the deep and symbolic meanings of places in our lives reflects an attitude that is closed to the possibilities of the world and of human beings. This attitude "involves a leveling down of the possibilities of being, a covering-up of genuine responses and experiences by the adoption of fashionable mass attitudes and actions. The values are those of mediocrity and superficiality" (Relph, p. 80).

Tourism is a powerful homogenizing influence on the environment that leads to placelessness, according to Relph (1976). The creation of sites for tourists can lead to the destruction of the placeness of the local landscape and its replacement by "conventional tourist architecture and synthetic landscapes and pseudo-places" (p. 93). Relph referred to historical sites such as reconstructed pioneer villages and restored castles as the "plastic past" (p. 103). Such re-creations have no experiential history. Historical accuracy may or may not be present, but the reality of lived experience across time and space ("space-time depth" [Rowles, 1991 p. 266]) is absent. Other ways that placelessness is demonstrated is in the gigantism of skyscrapers and other huge structures that lack a human scale, in commercial developments and strip malls that offer only uniformity of place, and in the instability and impermanence that stems from places undergoing continuous redevelopment or urban renewal.

Rowles (1991) proposed that we occupational therapists have often reduced place to placelessness in our therapy; we have ignored our clients' experiences of being in place by our strong emphasis on doing and performance in therapy. In effect, because we focus so strongly on the performance aspects of occupation, we have relegated place to the position of a backdrop in a play, giving it only superficial and casual attention as we spotlight the action in the scene. Rowles is concerned that we have ignored the contributions of place to people's identities and well-being and have underestimated the importance of the meanings and values that underlie the environments in which people live. As he stated more recently, "The fledgling discipline of occupational science might usefully focus on developing deeper insight into the evolving *rapprochement* of person and place in the search for meaning" (2008, p. 127).

Even in the 1970s, Relph (1976) expressed apprehension about the power of the forces of placelessness in our world today. In his view, human beings have a deep need for associations with significant places, and if we allow placelessness to go unchallenged, "then the future can only hold an environment in which places simply do not matter" (p. 147). In their own way, the sisters in the previous case example challenged the therapist to overcome her initial view of their home as merely space—placeless—and to, instead, attend to the meaning of their home and their sense of place within it. Relph would definitely applaud their efforts and the responsiveness of the therapist.

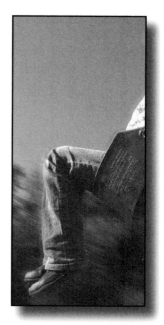

## A Place to Call Home

What, then, is the meaning of *home* as space and place? Home has been described as the place that provides the "centered-ness" of a person's life (Buttimer, 1980, p. 170). Buttimer described home as integral to the reciprocal movements of our lives:

> like breathing in and out, most life forms need a *home* and *horizons of reach* outward from that home … rest and movement, territory and range, security and

adventure ... centering suggests an ongoing life process—the breathing in and bringing home which is a reciprocal of the breathing out and reaching toward horizon. (pp. 170-171)

Sometimes we use the word *home* to refer to more expansive domains of our lives; for example, we might speak of being "at home" in the world, or in our own country, region, state, city, or neighborhood. But it seems, most commonly, we use the term home to refer to the specific dwelling in which we reside, day in and day out—the house that is our home, the place where we belong.

In Rowles' paper, "A Place to Call Home" (1987), he described the multiple meanings of home—as a symbol of continuity and connection between past, present, and future; as an extension of the self; as a place offering security and a sense of belonging; as a place of refuge or retreat; as a symbol of social identity; as a place in which we feel a sense of competence, order, and control; as a symbol of social status; as a symbol of independence; and as a "fulcrum" of all "outgoing" and "incoming" (p. 340). Others have researched interesting specific experiences related to home, such as Steward's (2000) study on the meaning of home to individuals who have home offices and Baldursson's (2004) exploration of the experience of "at-homeness" or feeling at home.

When we move from a home, especially one we have known for many years, we are dealt some wrenching blows to our sense of continuity and connection and our sense of self. It takes a while to establish a new sense of belonging, of order and control, of social identity, of at-homeness in the new place. The home we left gradually loses its sense of home for us, and the house we move into gradually takes on homelike characteristics.

We made such a move a few years ago, leaving behind the home we had known for almost 25 years. At some point on one of the many days that we spent sorting and packing, I remember finding our college-aged daughter, sitting quietly by herself at the top of the basement stairs in the only home she had ever known; with tears streaming down her cheeks, she looked up at me and said, "I was just remembering how we used to roller-skate in the basement."

Rowles calls such memories "autobiographical insideness" (1987, p. 341). Autobiographical insideness stems from the memories and sense of self that emanate from the spaces and artifacts maintained within the home. "Both the residence itself and the possessions it contains may serve as a museum of life history, the physical manifestations of a path traversed" (p. 341). The memories of our own childhoods, our children's play experiences, and the places where those experiences occurred provide a sense of connectedness for all of us to our own unique history. As Rowles reminds us, at every point in our lives, "we inhabit and are defined by a particular location and a particular time. ... Through the process of habitation, each location leaves its mark on us and, at the same time, becomes imbued with significance as a component of our ongoing life story" (2008, p. 129).

## *In the Corner of the Kitchen*

In my own childhood home, we had a rather remarkable feature that linked the house to us as a family. In one corner of the kitchen, beside the molding for the door that opened into the garage, was a sort of homemade version of a growth chart; all three children in the family, plus all visiting cousins, plus ultimately my parents' grandchildren and even great-grandchildren were represented at multiple points on the chart. For me, there was "Betty" at 3 years, 4 years, and every year after that up until age 17; each measurement was recorded in pencil with a small horizontal line and notation of my name and my age.

Problems arose when it came time to repaint the kitchen because these measurements were written directly on the wall; how could the "chart" be preserved for continued use? Eventually, we had a long board installed on hinges attached to the molding; we could paint the board the same color as the newly painted kitchen, and the hinges allowed us to either have the board closed and covering the growth chart, or swung open so that the chart was exposed, untouched, and available for adding new measurements. Over the years, that wall provided many moments of pleasure, amazement, and a strong sense of history for each of us as, from time to time, we paused to find our own or others' names on the chart.

We sold that house in 1991 after both of my parents died; no one from my family has lived there since then. But the hinged board and the pencil marks on the wall are still in the kitchen corner. The current owners had not known about the growth chart when they bought the house; they came upon the chart by chance one day as they were doing some redecorating. They were tremendously excited about their "find" and wanted to keep the hinged board and the chart on the wall intact. One might ask "Why?" since the penciled measurements are by this time somewhat smudged and the strip of original paint under the board is decidedly dingy. Further, the wall of names obviously could not be a place memory for these people who were so new to the house and who were not part of our family. Yet, I think, the names on the wall act like a living history to them, giving the house a sense of lived experience over time and space (i.e., Rowles' space–time depth). The growth chart helps to create a sense of place in the house. Even for the new owners, it helps transform the house into a home.

## Links Between People and Home

Rubinstein (1989) proposed three basic processes that link people to the home environment. The first, a *social-centered process*, is "the *ordering* of the home environment based on a person's version of sociocultural rules for domestic order" (p. S47). The way each of us makes order in a home is culturally based, including the kind of furniture we have and use, the placement of the furniture, how and where we store our possessions, our expectations for privacy within the home, expectations for cleanliness and neatness, and so forth. The importance to the two sisters of maintaining usual everyday routines in the previous occupational therapy case example is a striking illustration of the high priority attached to domestic order in some households.

The second process that links people to the home environment is the *person-centered process;* this process encompasses the expression of our life course through the features of the home environment. Personalization of the home and other expressions of the self in the home are part of the person-centered process. The growth chart in the kitchen was surely part of this process. All expressions of personal interest and personal history in a home—choice of colors in the décor, choice of paintings and art objects, displays of collections, choice of magazines and books, style of furnishings, the presence of family heirlooms, photographs on display, as well as plantings in the garden—are part of the person-centered process. When new owners move into a home and immediately begin to redecorate, they are expressing this need to personalize their house, and this personalization is one step in the process of transforming the house into a home.

The third process that links person to home is the *body-centered process*; the relationship of the body to the environmental features of the home is of central concern in this process. Manipulating the home environment to accommodate changing physical capacities, such as replacing the crib with a single bed for the developing child or installing a grab bar by the bathtub to accommodate increasing balance problems, represents the body-centered process. The occupational therapist in the case example of the home visit put her highest priority on this process, until she listened more closely and realized that the family's priority was on the social-centered concerns of the house—their perspective of domestic order.

## Homeyness

Rubinstein's (1989) three processes represent one way to describe elements of place as they relate to home. Another way to capture the meaning of home is to examine the concept of "homeyness" (McCracken, 1989). McCracken described homeyness in North America in three ways—as physical, symbolic, and pragmatic. The *physical properties* of homeyness include certain colors (an all off-white living room is *not* homey); the materials used for the walls (outside and inside); fabrics used for the furniture and furniture styles; the presence of personally significant objects, plants or flowers, seasonal decorations; architectural details such as wood-beamed ceilings and built-in bookshelves (filled with books).

The *symbolic properties* of a homey house are those intangibles that reflect the home's personality. For example, grand and elegant is not homey; small and informal is homey. The symbolic property of embracing is particularly interesting to me. The embracing aspect of a home relates to its aura of enclosure; fences, walls, shrubbery, an overhanging roof line, awnings, small windows, books lining the walls inside, arrangements of paintings and photographs on the walls, and furniture arrangements within the rooms that foster a sense of intimacy all contribute to the embracing property of a house. McCracken (1989) likened the embrace of a house to the embrace of a parent, and he felt that the embracing characteristics of a house are directly related to the fashioning of the family that lives inside.

Finally, by *pragmatic properties*, McCracken (1989) refers to homeyness as an enabling context, a status corrector, a marketplace corrector, or a modernity corrector. For example, as an enabler, homeyness creates "the stage on which all of the various domestic enactments of self and family can be undertaken" (p. 175). As a status corrector, homeyness sends a message that counteracts the demands of the competition for status that is present in much of society. To strive for homeyness can be like a protection for people "from the intrusions and demands of the designer, the marketer, and the showy neighbor" (p. 177). Homeyness is beyond elegant, expensive, modern, impressive, showy, upscale—all those inherently competitive characteristics. Yet homeyness is a very positive and desirable element of an abode.

Rowles (1987) suggested that "the need for a home is a fundamental human imperative" (p. 339), a place of control and order in a world of chaos. When home is viewed as the fulcrum of one's life, as providing the centered-ness of daily existence, as a source for autobiographical insideness, then the primacy of home as space and place in people's lives becomes apparent. At least in Western culture, having a home *is* a fundamental imperative, and understanding the meaning of home is one important way to understand the shape of people's lives, their identities, and their everyday occupations.

## At Home in an Institution

To many people, the space and place of institutions represent the absolute antithesis of home and homeyness. Institutions tend to be large, not diminutive. They tend to be filled with furnishings and objects that offer no variety in style or fabric and have little or no personal significance to the people who live there. The rules and policies of an institution contribute to a formality that precludes the comfort and ease of living at home.

By definition, an institution offers no autobiographical insideness to the individual who comes to live there, no history of lived experience over time and space. An individual in an institution is likely to remain an observer or a participant in the setting rather than becoming an integral part of the whole of the surrounding environment. The stage upon which all the domestic activities of self and family have been enacted—home—is gone.

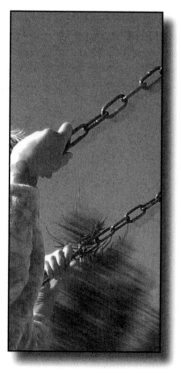

The powerful linking processes that exist between people and their homes are tenuous in an institution, if they exist at all. The ordering of the institutional environment is under someone else's control, the features of the environment do not reflect distinctive meanings and events from individual lives, and accommodation of the environment is governed by maximum accessibility guidelines, not by *individual* capacities.

The previous descriptions of what an institution is and isn't can be readily applied to long-term care settings, hospices, boarding schools, group homes, rehabilitation centers, retirement centers, and assisted living facilities. To be sure, an increased awareness of the dehumanizing effects of institutions has emerged in the last several decades. As early as 1961, Goffman coined the term *total institutions* and wrote his sensitizing analytical essays on the closed worlds of prisons, boarding schools, and mental hospitals. Almost a decade later, Illich (1970) wrote his book on the institutionalization of public education and the need to "deschool" society. Since then, institutional environments of all types have been changed or eliminated, as illustrated by the de-institutionalization movement in health care and the mainstreaming movement in education in the second half of the 1900s.

Homeyness within institutional settings has become a desirable sought-after attribute, now used by staff, for example, to project a positive image of the environment of residential facilities and nursing homes (Jacques & Hasselkus, 2004; Shield, 1990) and by researchers as a research variable (Thompson, Robinson, Graff, & Ingenmey, 1990). Personalization of the institutional environment and the creation of small communities within large institutions are viewed as important considerations. Being able to continue familiar routines and social roles is fostered through flexible rules, a variety of opportunities for involvement, and continued integration into the surrounding community (Hocking, 1996).

Focusing on one form of place-integration, Cutchin, Owen, and Chang (2003) have carried out research on the process of becoming at-home in an assisted living residence for older people. In developing at-homeness in this particular setting, new residents seem to be best served by being in a facility located in their own community and by engagement in meaningful social interaction and other activities with nonfamily members *within* the facility. The importance of within-institution activity and social relationship could be equated with building a semblance of autobiographical insideness. The residents are building memories and a sense of self in their new space.

The literature on the meaning of the institution, the impact of the institution on health and well-being, and modifications of institutions to diminish their potential deleterious effects is vast and beyond the scope of this chapter. Suffice it to say that the "total institutions" of Goffman's early 1960s are greatly reduced in numbers, and that settings of placelessness are being replaced with settings that offer at least a semblance of place that is meaningful.

## SPECIAL PLACES

The Mount Hope Cemetery in Rochester, New York, has burials of many prominent people, often with elaborate Victorian monuments of, well, monumental proportions! The cemetery office provides a guidebook for a walking tour of the grounds; using the booklet, one can visit the gravesites of various luminaries such as Frederick Douglass, renowned leader of the antislavery movement, and women's rights pioneer Susan B. Anthony. Once, while visiting our daughter in Rochester, we took the walking tour of Mount Hope, spending an hour or so walking among the ornate gravestones on which are recorded the barest of details of so many lives. Near the end of our tour, we finally found the grave of Susan B. Anthony. In contrast to so many other elaborate monuments, only a small square stone marked her grave. But the modest marker was not all that we found on her grave. Here also were coins, beads, and small pieces of jewelry—carefully laid on the base of the marker, presumably meant as symbols of respect, admiration, affection, recognition, and a sense of sisterhood—left by other visitors to this grave. Standing there, looking down at this unobtrusive gravesite with its own very personal tributes, we all felt that we were in a special place.

The world is full of special places. A special place is a place of heightened meaning and keen personal significance; whether or not a place is special is strictly personal. If I am in a place that is special to me, I cannot look at my companion and tell whether or not it is also special to him or her, unless their feeling of specialness is expressed in words or body language or actions. But, of course, that feeling of specialness usually *is* explicitly expressed in one way or another. For the three of us, standing there by Susan B. Anthony's grave, the sense of being in a special place was first expressed in our collective silent pause and then in exchanges of "Look at that!" kind of comments.

## Back to the Homeland

One kind of experience of a special place, particular to people whose ancestors emigrated from another country, is the experience of return to the homeland. When I stood inside the little church in north central Sweden where my mother's parents had been married in 1889, the strong sense of connection I felt to the grandparents whom I had never known was almost palpable. When we searched the back roads on Bodmin Moor in Cornwall and finally found the ruinous stone buildings that constituted the ancestral farm in my husband's mother's family, we were compelled to stop, smell the smells, see everything, touch the stones, and think about our connection to that special place.

Suzanne Bunkers' autobiographical account of her search for the life story of her great-great-grandmother describes the author's journey to her ancestral homeland of Luxembourg (1996). On her return to Luxembourg City in 1994, she wrote:

> When I come here, the tears start to flow. When I see the Luxembourg Cathedral of Notre Dame, I am overcome by a feeling that I can't explain. When I sit in the central square and realize that so many of my ancestors had to leave Luxembourg and could never come back, I feel so incredibly lucky to be here. I have the ability to be in a place that they no doubt longed for but could never see again. (p. 214)

Anyone who engages in family history research has experienced something similar to what Suzanne Bunkers describes in her autobiography. In some ways, genealogy is really the collection of special places—at home and abroad. Family history imbues certain sites and places with personal meaning and gives them space-time depth. Many of these sites become special places that one wants to visit again and again. And sometimes the tears flow—again and again.

## In a Room of One's Own

In 1929, Virginia Woolf wrote two papers, that were later expanded and combined into her timeless publication on women's intellectual and spiritual restriction in the modern world—*A Room of One's Own*. My "take" on the sometimes witty and always poignant writings in this book is that Woolf's use of the word *room* can be interpreted literally to mean a room of one's own *in a house* or symbolically as a place of personal meaning and influence in one's own life and world. Either kind of room, when it exists, can be a special place in a woman's world since women's lives have for so long been defined by the men with whom they associate. All people who feel the need for rooms of their own ought to be able to have one—a special place in which their individual humanity is honored and in which they can realize their own potential for meaningful involvement in the world.

Much more recently, another book with an almost identical title, *A Room of Her Own*, has been published. The author, Chris Casson Madden (1997), wrote about women who have created personal spaces within their homes or workplaces—a bedroom, an office, or even just a corner of a larger room. Madden's book seems to be a modern version of Woolf's essay, with an interpretation of "room" as a very personal physical space of retreat and comfort. Its characteristics are much the same as those that make up the concept of homeyness.

In her research on the work of scholars, Pierce (1996) described "the spaces of a scholar's work" (p. 133)—their offices—at home, at universities, in libraries, in laboratories. At my university, professors can reserve carrels at the library for the academic year. These small secure library spaces serve as hiding places for faculty, providing a space for work that is (potentially) beyond the reach of the telephone, the knock on the door, the E-mail messages. To the scholars in Pierce's study, the aesthetics of their offices on campus were usually regarded as important. In my own department, each faculty member has given at least some thought and attention to the décor of his or her office space—hanging posters, pictures, or framed copies of awards and degrees and other symbols of recognition on the walls; putting an attractive colorful rug on the bland tile floor to soften and liven up the room; displaying mementos of travels to meetings and conferences on top of the bookshelf or pinned to the bulletin board; putting plants on the windowsill; taping interesting clippings or pictures to the office door.

For the scholars in Pierce's study, in addition to their offices on campus, "the attainment of a satisfactory home office seemed to be a relished career milestone" (1996, p. 133). I have described the keen pleasure I found in the completion of the planning and refurbishment for my workspace at home in Chapter 9 in this book.

## Children's Experience of Place

In preparation for writing this chapter, I visited several of the libraries on campus, scanning potential resources related to space and place. One day I found my way to the library of the Department of Geography, home department of Yi-Fu Tuan, one of the humanistic geographers whom I quote and cite rather extensively in this chapter as well as others. The geography library is in one of the most historic and interesting buildings on campus—Science Hall. A big looming building of dark red brick, Science Hall has towers and turrets, stained glass windows and ceramic tile floors, and more nooks

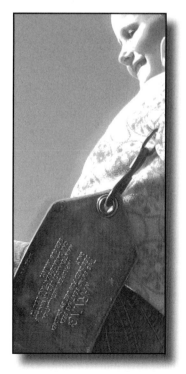

and crannies than you can possibly imagine. After climbing two flights of outside steps up to the massive front door, and then climbing more steps from the front door to the first floor hallway (a nightmare of inaccessibility), I followed the signs and climbed one more flight of stairs to the library on the second floor. And I struck gold.

I found a book published in 1979, describing a study with the title *Children's Experience of Place*. The author, Roger Hart, studied children and the development of children's experiences of place. Hart's purpose was to describe children's spatial behavior and land use, "while at the same time discovering their knowledge of, and feelings for, places in their environment" (p. 13). To study children and their spatial behavior, Hart lived for 2 years in a small New England town. He identified two clusters of children aged between 4 and 11 years and gradually got to know the children and their families, enlisting their willingness to allow him to observe their behaviors and engage them in a variety of space-related activities for the 2 years of the study.

As I read the various chapters of this study, I found myself flooded with memories of my own childhood experiences of place. My description of the swing at the start of this chapter was the direct result of my reading of Hart's (1979) research. Hart stated, "All children have an urge to explore the landscape around them, to learn about it, to give order to it, and to invest it with meaning—both shared and private" (p. 3). He mapped the "ranges" of movement about the neighborhood and community of the children in his study, and develops a typology for each age group consisting of (a) free range, (b) farthest distances of free range, (c) farthest distances of "with permission" ranges, and (d) farthest distances of ranges "with permission and with other children." He described children's paths and shortcuts, where they go on tricycles and where they go on bicycles. Then he shifted to describing the children's scary places, dangerous places, highly valued places, secret places, favorite places, magic places, summer places, and winter places. Hart delved into and elaborates on his discovery that all children *create* places that are "house-like"; in other words, in one way or another, children make a "house" or enclosure—in the woods, in the back yard, under the stairs, in a tree, in the leaf pile, in a corner of the playroom, in the snowdrifts.

As a geographer, Hart's (1979) purpose for the study was to gain understanding of children's spatial behaviors and needs as related to the design of neighborhoods and communities. When I was talking enthusiastically about this study with a colleague, she shared with me a quote from a book on gardening, in which the author, Michael Pollan (1991), described his "first garden"—a secret place between the backyard lilacs and the neighbor's wooden fence—created by him at the age of 4 years as a refuge from the adults in his world. Michael's "garden" is a lovely example of a child's experience of place.

> My first garden was a place no grown-up ever knew about, even though it was in the backyard of a quarter-acre suburban plot. Behind our house in Farmingdale, on Long Island, stood a rough hedge of lilac and forsythia that had been planted to hide the neighbor's slat wood fence. My garden, which I shared with my sister and our friends, consisted of the strip of unplanted ground between the hedge and the fence. I say that no grown-up knew about it because, in an adult's picture of this landscape, the hedge runs flush against the fence. To a 4-year-old, though, the space made by the vaulting branches of a forsythia is as grand as the inside of a cathedral, and

there is room enough for a world between a lilac and a wall. Whenever I needed to be out of range of adult radar, I'd crawl beneath the forsythia's arches, squeeze between two lilac bushes, and find myself safe and alone in my own green room. (p. 9)

Pollan has given us a child's version of a room of one's own.

A recent news article about a small neighborhood park near my home helped me think further about children's play and play spaces (Gabriel, 2009). Glenwood Park is a gem of a natural space with glens, rock outcroppings, trees of all sizes, and places to climb and hide. The park had been more or less unused for many years. As Gabriel wrote in the article, "Free play in nature is a vanishing pastime"; in fact, today's children often view the unstructured outdoors as somewhat fearsome. This past summer, however, due to a concerted effort by a few individuals in the neighborhood, the park is more and more being seen as a safe and friendly place—a welcoming space for some free-range childhood play. For example, a creative person in the neighborhood stuck a sign in a pile of dead branches in the park that said, "These materials may be used in the park for forts and other structures." In response to these efforts to make the park an inviting place for play, Gabriel was inspired to take her grade school son's birthday party there for a couple hours. A collective shout of "Yeah" went up from the group at first glimpse of the hand-lettered sign, and they were off and running with the fort building immediately. She had brought a few games along in case the boys got bored—but they never did.

Of course the homeland, a room of one's own, and children's places are just a very few examples of the special places in this world that each one of us has. These are special places in which we engage in the occupations of our choice. The characteristics of a special place are usually, perhaps always, linked strongly to the kinds of occupations that occur there; each special place is a setting for particular kinds of occupations and behaviors. Recognizing this intimate relationship enriches our understanding of the meanings of space, place, and occupation.

## A GEOGRAPHY OF HEALTH

When the emphasis in a profession is on the relationship between health and space and place, the field may be referred to as *medical geography* or *the geography of health* (Kearns, 1993; Moss, 1997). One example of research from medical geography is the study on planned home births carried out by Abel and Kearns (1991). The women in the study reported a greater sense of "healthiness" when the birth experience took place in the home, and their positive feelings about their homes were heightened by this choice. The reemergence of planned home births in recent years is one example of a place-centered change represented in health care. Abel and Kearns speculated that these feelings about the home as a place for birthing stemmed in part from the women's rejection of the use of medicalized institutional environments for what they perceived to be an "ordinarily healthy life event" and, further, that "large metropolitan hospitals are perceived by some as displacing patients from their familiar settings and bringing to birth feelings of placelessness" (p. 143). In the home birthing study, the importance of the women's experiences of place clearly extends into their conceptions of health and health care.

Another example of research from medical geography is the research by Moss (1997) in which she studied the way older women living with arthritis negotiate space in their home environments. Moss conceptualized the home space as an environment shaped by the domestic labor and social relations that occur there. She used the term *relational space* (p. 24) to convey space as inseparable from its social dimensions. In a variation of this concept of relational space, Warin, Baum, Kalucy, Murray, and Veale (2000) studied the way community health centers contribute to "the broader health of communities by acting as gathering places and arenas of information exchange" (p. 1865). The authors concluded that the relational experiences associated with the time and space of the centers had a positive effect on the health status of the patients as well as the community by diminishing barriers to health services, increasing community participation, providing safe places for social interaction and strengthening people's sense of belonging to community and place.

Within our own occupational therapy literature, Wood, Womack, and Hooper (2009) explored relationships among quality of life, activity patterns, and the environments of two special Alzheimer care units—one private, small, and homelike, the other larger and more like a "traditional nursing home environment" (p. 339). Unexpectedly, the results showed no difference between the facilities on quality of life indicators, and neither care unit supported meaningful daily time use patterns in the residents. The transactional nature of the phenomenon of people, space, and therapeutic environments is complex; our understandings are still rudimentary.

Finally, in another variation on relational space, Rowles' study of the surveillance zone as meaningful space (1981) remains a classic in the literature on space and aging. Rowles explored the meaning of the surveillance zone of older people, defined as the space within the visual field of home. He found that the extent and qualities of the surveillance zones that he studied contributed to the well-being of the older home owners in the small Appalachia community in his study in at least three ways: by facilitating the maintenance of practical and social support from neighbors, by providing an ongoing source of environmental participation, and by supporting a sense of identity for the old person. Often by the use of just a single window, individuals experienced visual participation in the space outside their homes—watching and being watched. Rowles concluded that, for the older person, the surveillance zone is a symbol of continuity and continuing participation in the world.

Many of the concerns and research interests of the field of medical geography are closely allied to the concerns of occupational therapy practice and to the research interests of occupational science. The meanings of space and place, and how those meanings help shape the daily occupations and well-being of individuals in their everyday worlds, are of paramount importance to both fields. Each field has literature and research activity that can enrich and fertilize the other. I think increased awareness and recognition of each other and increased opportunities for combined efforts in research and practice will ultimately be of benefit to both.

# REFERENCES

Abel, S., & Kearns, R. A. (1991). Birth places: A geographical perspective on planned home birth in New Zealand. *Social Science & Medicine, 33*, 825-834.

Baldursson, S. (2004). The nature of at-homeness. Retrieved from http://www.phenomenology-online.com/articles/baldursson.html.

Bunkers, S. L. (1996). *In search of Suzanna*. Iowa City: University of Iowa Press.

Buttimer, A. (1980). Home, reach, and the sense of place. In A. Buttimer & D. Seamon (Eds.), *The human experience of space and place* (pp. 166-187). New York, NY: St. Martin's Press.

Casey, E. S. (1987). *Remembering: A phenomenological study*. Indianapolis, IN: Indiana University Press.

Casey, E. S. (1996). How to get from space to place in a fairly short stretch of time. In S. Feld & K. Basso (Eds.), *Senses of place* (pp. 13-52). Santa Fe, NM: School of American Research Press.

Cutchin, M. P. (2003). The process of mediated aging-in-place: A theoretically and empirically based model. *Social Science & Medicine, 57,* 1077-1090.

Cutchin, M. P. (2005). Spaces for inquiry into the role of place for older people's care. *Journal of Clinical Nursing, 14,* 8b, 121-129.

Cutchin, M. P., Owen, S. V., & Chang, P. J. (2003). Becoming "at home" in assisted living residences: Exploring place integration processes. *Journal of Gerontology: Social Science, 58B,* S234-S243.

de Certeau, M. (1984). *The practice of everyday life*. Berkeley: University of California Press.

Dickie, V. A., Cutchin, M. P., & Humphry, R. (2006). Occupation as transactional experience: A critique of individualism in occupational science. *Journal of Occupational Science, 13,* 83-93.

Dunn, W., Brown, C., & McGuigan, A. (1994). The ecology of human performance: A framework for considering the effect of context. *American Journal of Occupational Therapy, 48,* 595-607.

Erikson, A., Karlsson, G., Söderström, M., & Tham, K. (2005). A training apartment with electronic aids to daily living: Lived experiences of persons with brain damage. *American Journal of Occupational Therapy, 58,* 261-271.

Fänge, A., & Iwarsson, S. (2005). Changes in ADL dependence and aspects of usability following housing adaptation: A longitudinal perspective. *American Journal of Occupational Therapy, 59,* 296-304.

Gabriel, M. E. (2009, June 20). Back to nature: Getting kids to rediscover the great outdoors. *The Capital Times*, Retrieved from http://www.madison.com/toolbox/index.

Gitlin, L. N., Corcoran, M., & Leinmiller-Eckhardt, S. (1995). Understanding the family perspective: An ethnographic framework for providing occupational therapy in the home. *American Journal of Occupational Therapy, 49,* 802-809.

Goffman, E. (1961). *Asylums*. Garden City, NY: Doubleday & Company.

Graesch, A. P. (2004, May). Notions of family embedded in the house. *Anthropology News*.

Hart, R. (1979). *Children's experience of place*. New York, NY: Irvington Publishers.

Helfrich, C., Kielhofner, G., & Mattingly, C. (1994). Volition as narrative: Understanding motivation in chronic illness. *American Journal of Occupational Therapy, 48,* 311-318.

Hocking, C. (1996). Promoting occupational performance for entering residents in long-term care. *Physical & Occupational Therapy in Geriatrics, 14,* 61-73.

Illich, I. (1970). *Deschooling society*. Evanston, IL: Harper & Row.

Jacques, N., & Hasselkus, B. R. (2004). The nature of occupation surrounding dying and death. *OTJR: Occupation, Participation and Health, 24,* 44-53.

Kearns, R. A. (1993). Place and health: Towards a reformed medical geography. *The Professional Geographer, 45,* 139-147.

Langer, S. (1953). *Feeling and form.* New York, NY: Charles Scribner's Sons.

Law, M., Cooper, B., Strong, S., Stewart, D., Rigby, P., & Letts, L. (1996). The person-environment occupation model: A transactive approach to occupational performance. *Canadian Journal of Occupational Therapy 63,* 9-23.

Leibrock, C. (2000). *Design details for health: Making the most of interior design's healing potential.* New York, NY: Wiley.

Madden, C. C. (1997). *A room of her own: Women's personal spaces.* New York, NY: Random House.

Mattingly, C. (1994). The concept of therapeutic "emplotment." *Social Science & Medicine, 38,* 811-822.

McCracken, G. (1989). "Homeyness": A cultural account of one constellation of consumer goods and meanings. In E. C. Hirschman (Ed.), *Interpretive consumer research* (pp. 168-183). Provo, UT: Association for Consumer Research.

Moss, P. (1997). Negotiating spaces in home environments: Older women living with arthritis. *Social Science & Medicine, 45,* 22-33.

Pierce, D. (1996). The work of scholars. In R. Zemke & F. Clark (Eds.), *Occupational science: The evolving discipline* (pp. 125-141). Philadelphia, PA: F. A. Davis.

Pierce, D., Munier, V., & Myers, E. T. (2009). Informing intervention through an occupational science description of infant-toddler interactions with home space. *American Journal of Occupational Therapy, 63,* 273-287.

Pohl, P. S., Froehlich-Grobe, K., McKiernan, B., Vacek, K. M., Donnelly, M., & Gaughan, J. F. (2006). Access to polling places in the 2004 presidential election: The experience of one metropolitan Midwestern city. *American Journal of Occupational Therapy, 60,* 404-408.

Pollan, M. (1991). *Second nature: A gardener's education.* New York, NY: Dell.

Relph, E. (1976). *Place and placelessness.* London, UK: Pion Limited.

Rowles, G. D. (1981). The surveillance zone as meaningful space for the aged. *The Gerontologist, 21,* 304-311.

Rowles, G. D. (1987). A place to call home. In L. L. Carstensen & B. A. Edelstein (Eds.), *Handbook of clinical gerontology* (pp. 335-353). New York, NY: Pergamon.

Rowles, G. D. (1991). Beyond performance: Being in place as a component of occupational therapy. *American Journal of Occupational Therapy, 45,* 265-271.

Rowles, G. D. (2000). Habituation and being in place. *Occupational Therapy Journal of Research, 20*(Suppl.), 52S-67S.

Rowles, G. D. (2008). Place in occupational science: A life course perspective on the role of environmental context in the quest for meaning. *Journal of Occupational Science, 15,* 127-135.

Rubinstein, R. L. (1989). The home environments of older people: A description of the psychosocial processes linking person to place. *Journal of Gerontology, 44,* S45-S53.

Sanford, J. A., Pynoos, J., Tejral, A., & Browne, A. (2002). Development of a comprehensive assessment for delivery of home modifications. *Physical & Occupational Therapy in Geriatrics, 20,* 43-55.

Seamon, D. (2002). Physical comminglings: Body, habit and space transformed into place. *OTJR: Occupation, Participation, and Health, 22*(Suppl. 1), 425-515.

Shield, R. R. (1990). Liminality in an American nursing home: The endless transition. In J. Sokolovsky (Ed.), *The cultural context of aging: Worldwide perspectives* (pp. 331-352). New York, NY: Bergin & Garvey Publishers.

Stegner, W. (1992). *Where the bluebird sings to the lemonade springs* (pp. 199-206). New York, NY: Random House.

Stevenson, R. L. (n.d.). The swing. In *A child's garden of verses* (p. 69). Chicago, IL: M. A. Donohue & Co.

Steward, B. (2000). Living space: The changing meaning of home. *British Journal of Occupational Therapy, 63,* 105-110.

Thompson, T., Robinson, J., Graff, M., & Ingenmey, R. (1990). Home-like architectural features of residential environments. *American Journal of Mental Retardation, 95,* 328-341.

Tuan, Y. F. (1977). *Space and place: The perspective of experience.* Minneapolis, MN: University of Minnesota.

Tyson, M. M. (1998). *The healing landscape: Therapeutic outdoor environments.* New York, NY: McGraw-Hill.

Warin, M., Baum, F., Kalucy, E., Murray, C., & Veale, B. (2000). The power of place: Space and time in women's and community health centres in South Australia. *Social Science & Medicine, 50,* 1863-1875.

Woolf, V. (1929). *A room of one's own.* New York, NY: Harcourt, Brace & World.

Wood, W., Womack, J., & Hooper, B. (2009). Dying of boredom: An exploratory case study of time use, apparent affect, and routine activity situations in two Alzheimer's special care units. *American Journal of Occupational Therapy, 63,* 337-350.

Woon, P. G. K. (1991). *Feng shui: The geomancy and economy of Singapore.* Singapore: Shinglee Publishers.

CHAPTER 4

# CULTURE AND OCCUPATION: THE EXPERIENCE OF SIMILARITY AND DIFFERENCE

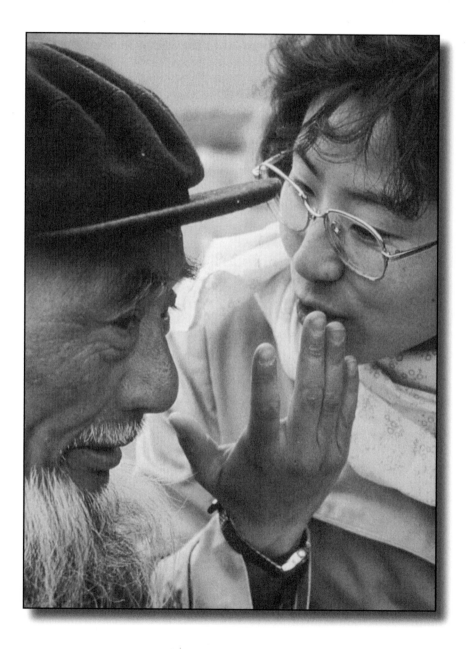

We learn and relearn who we are on the basis of our encounters with objects, ideas, and people—in short, with every different kind of "otherness."

Pollio, Henley, and Thompson (1997, p. 8)

The term *culture* has been used to refer to the patterns of values, beliefs, symbols, experiences, and learned behaviors shared by members of a group and passed from one generation to the next (Iwama, 2007; Krefting & Krefting, 1991; Rapoport, 1980). Geertz (1973) described culture as webs of significance, spun by human beings, the analysis of which is "an interpretive one in search of meaning" (p. 5). Ironically, although the word culture refers to shared beliefs, behaviors, and webs of significance, some have said that the only way to understand culture, especially as it relates to one's own habitus, is to appreciate the concept of "otherness" (Pollio, Henley, & Thompson, 1997; Whiteford & Wilcock, 2000). To recognize that something is "different" is to be able also to recognize what is similar.

## CULTURE AS SIMILARITY AND DIFFERENCE

On my first trip to Europe, I became very much aware of the "other" when I sat down to my first full-cooked English breakfast: two fried eggs, thick chunks of bacon, a grilled tomato, grilled mushrooms, fried bread, toast, marmalade, and coffee (cholesterol heaven!). This was not like breakfast at home. In Germany, a week later, breakfast consisted of brown soft-boiled eggs, slices of cheeses and cold meats, hard rolls, strawberry jam, juice, and coffee. When new to this kind of travel, a person suddenly realizes that breakfasts have certain predictable characteristics according to what country you are in but also that they are "different" from those at home. A consciousness of exactly what breakfast *is* at home emerges; we become aware that breakfast at home, too, has foods and customs that are predictable but both similar and different from those found in other countries. Mattingly and Beer (1993) stated, "Our own culture becomes much more visible in the face of a different culture" (p. 161).

Thus, what we are aware of in others reveals to us who *we* are. This phenomenon is similar to what Agar (1994) called "rich points"—those times in life during which we come up against a word, situation, or behavior that does not fit our own world. Each of us inhabits a cultural world. We may not be aware of our own worlds as cultural[1] but may, instead, think of our worlds as simply the way things are—as "normal." When we come up against a situation that we perceive as different, we may experience a rich point and come to realize that what we are accustomed to is only one way of being in the world, and that our own customs are likely to be experienced as *different* by someone else. Breakfast time offers just one of innumerable opportunities for us to experience rich points when traveling, to negotiate sameness and difference, and to recognize and come to understand the "other" at the same time that we gain understanding of ourselves.

---

[1]This ignorance of my own cultural ways of being in the world was brought home to me in the feedback I received from a colleague on an early draft of this chapter. To her, my own cultural perspective was "showing" in much of what I had written. I had recognized the Western cultural perspective in general, and even labeled it as such in several places in the chapter text. But she was able to see it at a deeper level in ways that, even when she pointed the sections out, were not obvious to me. We are, indeed, likely to be blind to our own deep cultural views.

Hasselkus, B. R.
*The Meaning of Everyday Occupation, Second Edition* (pp. 63-82).
© 2011 SLACK Incorporated

One could describe culture as the similarities and differences in people's life worlds, revealed in the rich points of life (Agar, 1994; Frank, 2000). The rich points in our lives are moments that can lead to a heightened awareness and appreciation of both our own culture and the culture of others; the more I understand the other (difference), the better I understand myself in my own habitat (the familiar). Occupation is a primary vehicle by which we experience rich points.

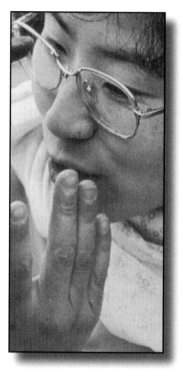

## Ethnocentrism

Lack of understanding and appreciation of the other is referred to as ethnocentrism. Ethnocentric people are those whose views of the world are circumscribed by the meaning of their own experiences. From an ethnocentric point of view, unfamiliar cultures are judged and defined only in comparison to what is familiar, often with the view that what is familiar is superior (Krefting & Krefting, 1991); "others" are recognized as different, but only in the sense that the difference is viewed as undesirable, grounded in ignorance, or even inferior.

A cousin in my family traveled mostly within the United States, but on one rare occasion, he and his wife ventured into the province of Quebec, Canada. Upon their return home, he openly expressed his irritation with the French-speaking people of Quebec; "Why don't they speak English?" I have been with tour groups of Americans in Europe when the need to change currency as we crossed the border from one country to another (a need now diminished by the adoption of the Euro in many countries) prompted sighs of exasperation and bewilderment; "Why can't they accept the U.S. dollar everywhere?" Both of these remarks represent ethnocentric points of view. I think such reactions to difference in others are rooted in a lack of awareness that our own worldview, too, is culturally shaped.

## The Deeper Threads

The examples above strongly link difference to identity—Canadian, American, European, English, German, or even simply "foreign." Agar (1994) stated that ethnocentrism is when an understanding of difference stops at the identity level. Rich points in a person's life can move him or her beyond the ethnocentrism of identity and difference to changes in consciousness that open up new ways of seeing and doing things. To move beyond ethnocentric thinking at a rich point in life, a person compares the difference he or she has just come up against with other differences present in the situation until "the deeper threads that tie the differences together" (Agar, p. 129) become visible for the first time. This concept of deep threads is akin to the webs of significance proposed by Geertz (1973). Agar's metaphor is of threads that tie differences together (of course threads also tie similarities together, but those threads are likely not the ones that reveal culture to us), and out of the threads emerges a pattern, and the pattern indicates coherence, and the coherence is—voilá—*culture*! "Whatever culture is, it shows patterns, the connections among different things" (Agar, p. 138).

Using Agar's framework of "deeper threads," it appears to me that my cousin is clearly seeing the situation in Quebec as composed of difference (people using a language that is different from his own) and identity (the people are Canadians). "Why don't they speak English?" But if we experience the rich point in a way that moves us beyond such ethnocentric thinking, we look deeper, we recognize many other differences imbedded in the situation, and we can begin to see some coherence among the threads, tying the differences together. The languages of the world are not simply sets of words or mechanisms that enable people to speak to one another. Languages are vivid representations of culture; Agar (1994) would say that language cannot exist without culture and culture cannot exist without language. So the difference represented by the non-English language spoken to my cousin in Quebec is much more than a bunch of unfamiliar words; the French language represents a different history and heritage, customs of relationship, political beliefs and ideas, mannerisms, modes of dress, and meal customs. Coherence exists across these differences, born of the deep threads of French and Canadian history, ancestry, life experiences, and political forces that tie these differences together. Why don't they just speak English? Because English is not who they are nor is it who they want to be. And language represents much more than simply calling a potato a potato rather than a pomme de terre. As Agar said in his discussion about language theory, language is connected "to the situations of its use" and words and sentences "sit in the context of the discourse that contains them" (p. 96). Language is not just about words and sentences, and meaning goes well beyond what the dictionary and rules of grammar offer.

Obviously, coming up against rich points in one's life does not eliminate difference. My cousin's perspective and the French-Canadian perspective about language remain different. But an openness to the many differences that exist in the situation, and subsequent new understandings about the deeper threads that tie those many differences together, can lead one to a heightened awareness and appreciation of both one's own culture and the culture of others.

## Culture Evolving

In addition to ethnocentrism, the reactions of my cousin and of my fellow travelers also reflect different, more recently evolving challenges to the concept of culture. The emphasis in new conceptualizations shifts from culture as the patterns or webs of shared meanings and experiences in people's lives to culture as it *restricts and inhibits* people's ways of seeing and doing in the world (see discussion in Ortner, 2006, pp. 107-128 regarding individual agency, determinism, and subjectivity). Patterns of behavior and beliefs are positioned in competition with each other; "cultures involve conflicting ways of thinking about and doing things" (Frank, 2000, p. 48). Defined in this way, we could say that my cousin's Midwestern cultural habitus restricted him from appreciating and valuing the differences represented by the people of Quebec who spoke French. His exasperation that they did not speak English reflects a competitive stance, a sort of "our way is *the* way" view of the world. The reactions of the tour group members to the differing currencies of European countries reflect a similar stance.

## Culture, Occupation, and Occupational Therapy

Patterns of beliefs and behaviors are strongly present in all the occupations of our everyday lives. The routines of our daily activities, the symbols and images found in our day-to-day surroundings, the priorities we set as we plan our days, our perceptions of what kinds of activities are "appropriate" as related to our community, country, gender, age, size, color, past experiences, religious upbringing, social relationships, obligations, and responsibilities—all of these phenomena constitute elements of culture in our occupational lives. In the words of Pollio et al. (1997), "What we experience is … never separate from the culture or language in which we live, talk, and act" (p. 8).

The importance of understanding and appreciating the cultural contexts of people's occupational worlds has gained recognition in recent years within occupational therapy and occupational science. In the United States, culture is included as an occupational therapy domain of practice in professional documents (American Occupational Therapy Association [AOTA], 2008). Fitzgerald (2000) and others (Iwama, 2005, 2007; Jungersen, 2002; Odawara, 2005), while recognizing recent increasing sensitivities to culture within occupational therapy, nevertheless urge us to continue to expand our understandings. As Iwama stated, culture speaks not only to "issues of diversity and inclusion but also to the creation of knowledge, theories, and the structures and contents of occupational therapy practices" (2007, p. 184). Iwama strongly proposed the need for therapists to "recognize the cultural construction of occupational therapy itself" (2005, p. 138), raising our awareness of the Western ideologies historically imbedded in our practice. Hammell (2009), too, reminded us that occupational therapy is both shaped by culture and is a culture itself. She cautioned us to be aware that occupational therapy assumptions and values (e.g., valuing independence and autonomy) reflect particular cultural perspectives and are not universal truths. To have cultural competence is to be able to reach beyond culture as represented in race and ethnicity and to look inward, challenging our own assumptions, values, and beliefs as individuals and as a health care profession.

Nor should culture be viewed as a static phenomenon—rather, culture is increasingly viewed as "emergent in the everyday interactions of individuals" (Bonder, Martin, & Miracle, 2004, p. 161). Beliefs, values, and patterns of behavior are ever changing and evolving, including across the time and interactions that take place during the therapy process (Odawara, 2005). In keeping with this dynamic view of cultural change, Dean proposed that, instead of striving for cultural competence, we recognize our *lack* of competence, aiming for "a state of mind in which we are interested and open, but always tentative about what we understand" (2001, p. 629). After all, how can we hope to attain competency of a phenomenon that is continually changing? As Black and Wells stated, "Cultural competency is a journey rather than an end" (2007, p. 31).

From an anthropological view, culture is what makes the experiences of life meaningful and culture is what gives intelligibility to what we do (DiGiacomo, 1999). If we accept the assumption that the cultures of our worlds are intimately intertwined with the meaning of occupation in our lives, then culture rises to what Iwama (2007) described as an "eminent place" in occupational therapy. Iwama suggests that the promise of occupational therapy in our world today is "to enable people from all walks of life to engage or participate in activities and processes that have value" (2007, p. 183). The importance of thinking more deeply about our sociocultural world and the concepts of similarity and difference is apparent.

# CULTIVATING THE SIMILAR IN OUR LIVES

Pick an event in your life—any event. Then begin to think about the event as a form of occupation—that is, as engagement in *doing*, as *being* in the world, as a reflection of *belonging*, and as *becoming* who we are (Hammell, 2004; Wilcock, 1998, 2006). Then think about the event as a *sociocultural* occupation—engagement that both shapes and is shaped by beliefs, symbols, rituals, routines, experiences, attitudes, institutional forces, and personal perceptions.

## The Visitation

When I was a teenager, the mother of one of my best friends died. Inexperienced as we were in matters of death, my friends and I somewhat nervously attended the visitation and ended up standing to one side, talking rather animatedly and loudly to each other. An adult friend of the family very soon came over to us and suggested quietly that our rather noisy behavior was not quite fitting for the occasion. Our behavior was out of sync with the expectations of the others who were there and were observing us; my friends and I were acting in a manner that was not within the parameters of behavior deemed appropriate in the setting.

Agar (1994) said that the experience of culture starts when you go "bottom-up"— when you are in a situation of differences that you don't know how to make sense of (p. 135). I think that my experience at the visitation was one of going bottom-up; my friends and I did not know how to make sense of the situation. We had little or no *frame* for the event (Agar's term), little to enable us to come up with expectations for what would take place, little to set limits around what to say and do. We had definitely come up against a rich point within our own cultural world.

The family friend helped to reveal just what the expectations *were* for our manner and appearance in that particular setting—we were expected to be not so loud, not so vivacious, more solemn. With her counsel ringing in our ears, my friends and I made a small start toward developing a frame for the visitation experience, toward seeing the many threads that both defined how this situation was different from others in our lives and that revealed how the differences in the situation were tied together to form some kind of coherent pattern within our own culture. I began to see the visitation in a new way, now more consciously aware that I was in a situation that was set apart from the ordinariness of daily life, from what was familiar to me up to this point in time.

In retrospect, I think that my friends and I had at first tried to pretend otherwise; we had, in effect, tried to ignore the "differences" in this situation by falling back on our accustomed ways of interacting with each other in other situations, relying on casual, animated conversation and joking around. The quiet word from the family friend put an immediate stop to that approach to the situation; we were not going to be able to pretend that being together at this visitation was pretty much the same as being together in other settings. We were going to have to acknowledge the differences and to try to make some sense out of all this unfamiliarity.

## The Threads of Difference

The differences that I came up against at the visitation were many and complex. Perhaps the first difference was revealed when I realized that this situation had its own very specific guidelines for human conduct. Social interactions were part of the occasion, but only certain types of social exchanges were acceptable. The visitation was in a funeral home, not a church or temple, yet I observed that some visitors carried out religious rituals such as kneeling at the casket and saying the rosary. A ritualized sequence of actions characterized the visitation, with visitors entering the room and proceeding to sign the guest book and pick up a memorial program; getting in line to express sympathy to the family members in words and with physical gestures such as crying, hugging, giving pats on the back, handshaking, and hand holding; standing silently for a few moments next to the casket (or for some this was the moment of kneeling and praying); and then, having reached the end of the most ritualized elements of the visitation, moving quietly out and about the room and talking informally to other people who were in attendance. So, although many occupational elements of the visitation event were familiar to me from other contexts in my life—signing a guest book, exchanging social greetings, carrying on conversational interactions, saying a prayer, being dressed up (an aspect of the occasion that I have not even mentioned but one that has many event-specific guidelines and expectations)—all also contained aspects of speech, manner, and appearance that were different from those of the more ordinary aspects of my daily life. These differences functioned as symbols in which the meanings of the ritual of the visitation were "stored" (Geertz, 1973, p. 127).

## The Webs of Significance

At this point you, the reader, may be already aware that I have only marginally addressed the most dramatic difference of all—the difference represented by the presence of a dead body. At a visitation, the existence of death in our lives is undeniable; the dead body in the room cannot be ignored, the room is a place of death (Malinowski, 1992). Gubrium and Holstein (2000) have said that in dying and death, "the body seems to explode with meaning, perhaps more so than at any other time of life" (p. 8). We are awed by death's presence; its significance is huge. Accordingly, the webs of significance that we spin around this phenomenon are many and deep. As Geertz stated, "That which is set apart as more than mundane is inevitably considered to have far-reaching implications for the direction of human conduct" (1973, p. 126). Faced with this extraordinary event, we turn to religion, the comfort of prescribed ritualized actions, the gathering of friends and family, physical expressions of caring and closeness, certain modes of dress, certain modes of speech, and demonstrations of emotion in an effort to express the deep differences between this event and other events of life and to infuse the event with coherence.

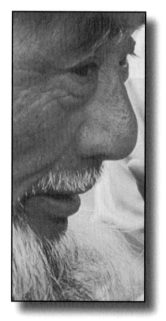

Mattingly and Beer (1993) made the observation that:

> We seem to need a way to identify and understand one another not only as individuals but also as members of larger groups that have certain characteristics in common. Culture is one term we use to locate ourselves and others as belonging to recognizable groups. (p. 157)

In our need to understand one another as members of larger groups with common characteristics, we cultivate patterns of behaviors, and out of the patterns eventually comes familiarity. Paradoxically, the familiar, thus, arises from differences. In this way, we become more comfortably situated as members within our own culture—belonging to a recognizable group.

The cultural aspects of any life situation, however, are reflected in much more than the explicit behaviors of the social actors in the scenario. The *meanings* and *interpretations* of our actions and the actions of the others in the situation were also affected by the events at the visitation. Immediately upon being cautioned by the adult friend, I remember feeling acutely embarrassed by my behavior; also immediately, I internalized the judgment that laughter and loud talking in such a setting were not appropriate. Within a very few seconds, I shifted from being immersed in conversation with my friends and ignorant of the cultural expectations of those around me to being acutely aware of, accepting, and *highly valuing* the need to act differently. To act only in certain ways in this situation became significant for me; the behaviors of others at the visitation, the ritualized aspects of the situation, the word choices I heard in the conversations around me, the way people were dressed—all took on significance for me. Geertz's (1973) web of significance began to take shape and my own behaviors began to be shaped by these significances.

Not only did the embarrassment at the visitation affect my behavior and my values and beliefs at the time, but it also influenced the way I interpreted subsequent situations, affecting the values and priorities I brought to other visitations. Such cultural characteristics, gradually and continuously acquired, familiarized, modified, redefined, and shared with others across our lifetimes—culture emergent—are present in all of our occupational pursuits.

## Balancing the Similar and the Different

The social rules for behaviors in our everyday lives are part of the shared beliefs and shared webs of significance that make up our culture; they are also obviously part of the restrictions and conflicts imposed by culture. The tension arising from the delicate balance between culture as positive and enriching and culture as constraining and limiting is made evident by Kalekin-Fishman (1987) in her research on the kindergarten experience in Israel in the mid-1980s. Just as my behavior at the visitation was shaped by the family friend, the behavior of the children in Kalekin-Fishman's study was shaped and monitored by the kindergarten teacher and the aide. The teacher's control over the children's behaviors in the classroom ranged from partial to total, and the only space where teacher control was negligible was on the playground. Kalekin-Fishman referred to the kindergarten as a "group-oriented, patterned-activity place ... the structure invested in space and time by planned activities is the key to an understanding of the kindergarten experience" (p. 83). The children were, in effect, what Goffman (1956) would call "front stage" (p. 13) all day long except during recess; the obligation to put on a good performance by conforming to the expectations of the teacher and the aide became crucial to their very existence as children in their kindergarten culture.

It may soon become obvious when reading the report of the kindergarten study that the effort to conform, to do what others expect, will lead to acceptance and even praise by cultural authorities (teachers, aides), but that the same effort may also stifle and extinguish individuality and creative behavior. Harsh critics of schooling have claimed that "extinguishing" is exactly what occurs in Western educational systems (as well as in other cultural institutions; Ferguson, 1980; Illich, 1970). Suffice it to say that a worthy teacher of children recognizes that schooling offers knowledge and experiences that are both liberating and confining; children in kindergarten learn the ways of the culture, but they relinquish aspects of their own natural ways of exploring and learning about their world in the process.

## CULTIVATING DIFFERENCE IN OUR LIVES

Perhaps it goes without saying that, by cultivating the similar, we, at the same time, cultivate the difference—the "other." By defining one, we define both. In the micro-culture of the visitation, my noisy behavior put me temporarily in the category of an other. Now that I have learned what is the expected behavior at such occasions, I blend in by acting in ways that are familiar to those who are also present. At the same time, now I am uncomfortable if someone else at a visitation acts in a loud or boisterous manner. I have defined and accepted the differences between the visitation and other situations of life, and on the basis of those differences, certain patterns of behavior have now become expected, familiar, and acceptable. By default, I have also defined what is outside of the familiar pattern and, thus, unacceptable—the other. The child who is beginning to understand the expected behaviors of being in the kindergarten class begins also to recognize behaviors that are outside those expectations; "telling" on another child is perhaps a strategy used by children to affirm their own position in the culture and to identify and "rein in" persons who are acting outside the culture (Kalekin-Fishman, 1987). Coming over to me to have a quiet word at the visitation was a strategy that similarly affirmed one person's position in the culture and reined in another person who was acting outside the culture.

To some extent, we spend our lives drifting back and forth between being insiders and being outsiders, being the same and being different. At times, we may purposely and consciously adhere to familiar cultural ways of behaving in order to be insiders; at other times, we may purposely flaunt the familiar ways in order to emphasize our outsider-ness.

Being an outsider within one's own culture or in relation to a larger culture is not necessarily negative or undesirable. The positive aspect of outside-ness is the theme of a current theatrical production in the United States titled *Undesirable Elements*. The production is the brainchild of Ping Chong, a performance artist and playwright who was an artist-in-residence at the University of Wisconsin–Madison in 2001. Chong was quoted in a local newspaper article as saying:

> As an artist, I'm an outsider in American society. As an experimental artist, I'm an outsider in the art world. As a person of color, I'm an outsider; as an immigrant, I'm an outsider; as a gay man, I'm an outsider. It's the position that fate has allotted me, but it's a valuable position to be in, because I think every society should have a mirror held to it by the outsider. (Goff, 2001)

Chong's theatrical production involves six people telling stories of their lives; the focus is on diversity and its possibilities. The production has appeared many times in various locations throughout the country, but each performance is community specific, using local performers who are selected on the basis of an intensive interview with the artist. As one of the performers in Madison said, "What resonates for me is the common denominator of 'otherness'" (Wolff, 2001).

We are, all of us, the "other" at certain times and in certain ways in our lives. Our "otherness" can be a source of rejoicing, as can our "belongingness" within the familiar.

## STRUCTURING THE SIMILARITIES: ROUTINES, HABITS, AND RITUALS

In her book on the life of writing, Annie Dillard has the following to say about daily occupations:

> What then shall I do this morning? How we spend our days is, of course, how we spend our lives. What we do with this hour, and that one, is what we are doing. A schedule defends from chaos and whim. It is a net for catching days. ... Each day is the same, so you remember the series afterward as a blurred and powerful pattern. (1989, p. 32)

*Routines*, *habits*, and *ritual*s are three terms that are frequently used to describe repetitive, predictable patterns of behavior in daily life. Dillard (1989) said that such patterns defend our daily lives from "chaos and whim." One of my favorite writers, Yi-Fu Tuan, has said something similar: "... stability is a cultural achievement without which any sort of sane life is impossible. Routines are therefore to be respected" (1994, p. 151).

Both Tuan (1994) and Dillard (1989) are saying that routines, habits, and rituals offer us sources of cultural stability in an otherwise chaotic existence, and, without these sources of stability, we human beings could not survive. In keeping with this perspective and the theme of similarity and difference in this chapter, I would expand further to suggest that these behavioral patterns are occupations that offer us ways to ensure the presence of, and the structure for, the "familiar" in our daily lives. They are part of what enables us to identify and recognize ourselves *as* our selves, and to situate ourselves within our own culture.

*Habits* have been defined by Dewey (1957) as "an acquired predisposition to ways or modes of response" (p. 40) and by Clark (2000) as the "relatively automatic things a person thinks or does repeatedly" (p. 128S). Alternatively, Clark defined *routines* as "a type of higher-order habit that involves sequencing and combining processes, procedures, steps, or occupations" (p. 128S). In Clark's view, routines are more outcome-driven than habits; they denote what a person will do and what sequential steps will be taken, leading to specific outcomes and orderliness in daily life. Gallimore and Lopez (2002) referred to a habit or routine as "a compromise between what is desirable and what is practical ... culture defines what is an ideal routine" (p. 705). Finally, *rituals*, too, are characterized by repetition, order, and predictability and are embedded in our daily lives; but in addition to traits held in common with habits and routines, rituals are infused with drama and symbolism and meaning-centeredness (Crepeau, 1995). Myerhoff (1977) stated that participants in rituals have certain parts or roles to play, upon which the success of the ritual depends.

## Habits and Routines as Liberating

Tuan (1994) offers us a perspective of routines as important and positive forces in our lives. Clark (2000) suggests further that habits and routines actually enable us to live *enriched* lives and to experience enhanced periods of creativity and innovation by the fact that they "free the brain" from the work of attending to the repetitive concerns of people's daily lives; "In this way, creative and innovative thinking can be 'embroidered' on a background of habitual structure" (p. 129S). This is a way of conceptualizing habits and routines that is in sharp contrast to the views of habits as stultifying and restrictive; quite the opposite, habits and routines can also be thought of as freeing and liberating. As long as I am able to attend to my mundane daily needs by carrying out the almost automatic routines and habits that I have developed over the years, then I will have enough energy to pursue other more creative and unique occupations during my day.

We know this to be the case when we are not feeling well. If I have a bad headache or am otherwise ill, my energy and initiative are drained by the usually automatic activities of basic self-care and simply moving around the house. But, of course, illness is not the only event that can reduce our abilities to carry out daily activities in a habitual or routine manner. Several years ago I spent 7 weeks in Australia as a visiting professor at the University of Sydney. I was struck, during my first days in this new place and culture, by how much energy it took to just attend to my everyday needs. Every single appliance (stove, clothes washer and dryer, iron, TV, radio, garbage disposal, thermostat, telephone, electrical outlets) took some mental energy to figure out how it worked because each one was slightly different from what I was used to at home. Just to go in and out of the apartment building itself meant mastering the security system on the main door and the key system for the elevator. My first foray out and about the neighborhood took fierce concentration—finding the grocery store, post office, take-out restaurants, bakery, bank, drug store—and I was slightly terrified that the security

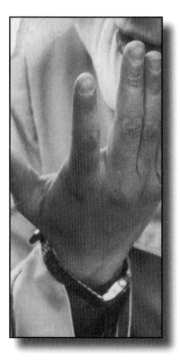

system would not let me get back into my apartment! The next day I had to tackle the hustle and bustle of the train system in order to ride many miles to the health sciences campus outside of Sydney.

Gradually, as those early days of my stay in Australia passed, more and more of my daily occupations became habitual and routine and, as the routinization set in, my energy level rose for more out-of-the-ordinary activities and adventures. In Clark's (2000) words, I gradually acquired a "background of habitual structure" that set my energies free to explore new and more challenging occupations. At the same time, I felt less and less like an outsider; I had mastered the routine demands of day-to-day living in Sydney, I felt like I belonged (albeit temporarily) to the working world of the city, and I had created a pattern of daily occupations that was now familiar and semiautomatic.

The resurrection of so much of the habitual nature of my daily occupations enabled me to once again experience a comparatively stable and familiar cultural world. The seemingly endless need to ask for directions, assistance, and explanations abated; I could get about with relative ease on my own. Ahhh, this was more like it! My sense of self-confidence, independence, and self-sufficiency—such strong elements of my American cultural ideology—were restored. Life felt more sane again.

## Rituals as Symbolic Meanings

But how does ritual fit into all this? Crepeau (1995) has said that a major difference between ritual and habits or routines is that rituals have strong symbolic meanings attached to them. Thus, although routinization is present in many rituals, born of their repetitious and predictable nature, symbolization is another prominent component, and the symbolization process is a "tool of meaning" (Fine, 1999, p. 23).

In my dissertation research on family caregivers who were caring for elderly family members in the community, I interviewed a daughter who was living with her mother and providing a high level of care for her mother all day and all night. This daughter–caregiver had a schedule of helpers who came in at certain times during the day to help with specific tasks, such as a friend who came from 5:00 p.m. to 6:00 p.m. every day—Monday through Sunday—to help lift her mother so she could use the commode and to help give her supper; this same friend also came again every evening at 9:00 p.m. for a short time, again to help lift her mother onto the commode and also to help put the mother to bed. One other friend and a paid helper alternated mornings on Monday through Friday, coming at 8:00 a.m. or 9:00 a.m. and staying into the early afternoon. On the weekends, a helper from the nurses' "pool" came in the mornings.

Built into these days were elaborate routines, or what I would call rituals, of activity such as the preparations this caregiver described for giving her mother medications:

> The sinimet pill is a mess if she doesn't swallow it. It gets on her. Well, we have her well protected ... we have an apron on her and then we have an extra towel, and then lately I put a double hand towel [over her chest] because it stains, this pill does. You'd have to bleach it every time.

The description of the steps taken to "protect" the bedding at night from getting "wet" was more elaborate:

> I pad her at night. What did we say—3, 4, 5, 6, 7 pads? And, uh, this protects the bed .... We put the double Chux down first, and then we put the

Pamper just flat and overlapping because she does quite a bit of rolling back and forth. Then we put on a fitted pamper; it's more absorbent than those cheaper flat ones." Interviewer: "Oh, does that go right on her then?" Caregiver: "No, just underneath, just flat. Then we take one of the flat ones and just tuck it under her, make sure that it's flat … So, um, the bed never gets wet, and that's what would make the work.

This daughter–caregiver was absolutely determined that her mother would continue to use the commode during the day (rather than rely on absorbent pads), even though, because of her own arthritis, she could not lift her mother without the help of another person. The scheduling of helpers during each day was timed to accommodate her mother's likely need to use the commode. For the most part, the scheduling of the helpers actually accomplished this goal; they were there when the commode was needed. The daughter referred to the rare occasions when her mother needed to go to the bathroom and no helper was present as "emergencies."

To me, the structured sequences of activities that this caregiver developed as part of her caregiving tasks, including the careful scheduling of helpers every day, all day long, represented something beyond routines and habits. For one thing, these sequences did not seem so much automatic or subconscious as purposeful and carried out with deliberation. They were sequences that this caregiver could describe in detail. When the planned routines did not "work," she described the situation as an "emergency." The successful completion of the weekly schedule and the daily routines seemed, in fact, to be vital to her need to feel that she was "managing." She worried terribly that the day might come when her friends and helpers might no longer be able to come; "I'm blessed with good friends, and my mother is blessed with enough capital to afford to pay the pool people, and I pray every night that that will continue." The roster of helpers and the elaborate routines such as those to keep the bed dry and to protect her mother's clothing *symbolized* control and manageability to her. The tremendous importance she placed on enabling her mother to continue to use the commode during the daytime—and the elaborate scheduling of helpers in order to do that—probably reflected the daughter's need to maintain a kind of normalcy of adult management of a bodily function for her mother; perhaps this helped her to continue to be able to think of her mother *as* her mother; perhaps her mother had strong wishes to be able to use the commode during the day related to her own sense of being an adult or her sense of what symbolized decency and dignity. Because of the strong symbolic nature of these activities, I would call them rituals.

## Rituals of Professional Health Care

In her research, Crepeau (1994) conceptualized the routines and patterns of interaction among psychiatric team members as ritual behavior. That the health care world is permeated with rituals surely defies argument. Those of us in the health care professions are usually very aware of the protocols for communication, deference, authority, control, and social interaction that exist in all health care settings. When rituals get interrupted, break down, or are disregarded, we experience uncomfortableness in the situation.

I experienced an awareness of the omission of a taken-for-granted ritual when my husband was hospitalized a few years ago for surgery to correct a potentially life-threatening problem. We awaited the visit from the surgeon the day after the surgery to hear the results of all the testing of the tissues surrounding the surgical site. It was with tremendous relief that we received the good news early that afternoon. The surgeon came, took a seat by the bed, and gave us news that was the best possible; I remember my exclamation, "Oh, Ed, we can get on with our lives."

Suddenly and surprisingly, while we were still deep in consultation with the surgeon, the head nurse on the surgical ward came into the room and interrupted our meeting to inform my husband that his bathrobe (brought from home) had been lost by the hospital laundry. She went on at some length about the measures she would take to try to track down the whereabouts of the robe and how she would keep us informed about the situation. The intimacy of our meeting with the surgeon was destroyed; he sat mute—forced to put his own planned conversation on hold and to wait silently while the nurse pursued the subject of the robe. I was at first astonished at what seemed like a major breach of protocol; a nurse, even a head nurse, should never interrupt a surgeon during his private consultation with a patient who has just had major surgery, especially about such a mundane topic as a misplaced bathrobe. Then I realized that the surgeon was wearing street clothes (thus not attired in one of the major symbols of his status) and that this was a big hospital where many doctors and nurses would not know each other; this head nurse probably thought that the person sitting beside the bed was a friend and visitor. If such was the case, then her interruption is not so surprising, as she might well consider her status to be higher than that of a visitor, giving her the right to interrupt.

In this nurse–surgeon scenario, a powerful ritual governing professional interactions in hospital settings had been disregarded. The expected ritualistic behavior among health professionals on the surgical ward holds tremendous symbolic meanings about the hierarchies of authority that exist, the professional status of the various personnel, the special regard and deference that is expected to be shown to certain members of the staff, the sacred nature of the doctor–patient consultation, and rules about who speaks first and to whom, and what forms of address are used (first name, last name with title). When the rules that govern the rituals of speech and interaction are broken, the occasion is not forgotten.

Cross-cultural differences represented in health care practices and health care beliefs can loom very large indeed, in contrast to the subtle bending of rules and protocols described in the example of the within-culture interaction between the head nurse and surgeon. In Anne Fadiman's (1997) superb and memorable account of the clash between a refugee Hmong family and the health care offered at a hospital in California, the physicians and nurses who tried to provide Western medicine for baby Lia Lee were frustrated to the extreme by the parents' refusal to follow the prescribed medication regimes and by the non-Western Hmong beliefs and

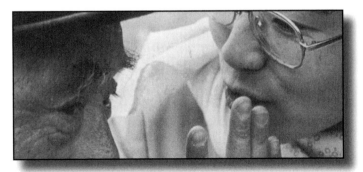

practices about health and the body. Baby Lia was hospitalized repeatedly for severe seizures, sometimes life threatening.

Fadiman (1997) stated that Hmong patients "never showed their doctors the kind of deference reflexively displayed by even their most uncooperative American patients" (p. 57). Reaching decisions about medical procedures that violated Hmong taboos—such as surgeries—often took hours; a hierarchy of consultations might include wives asking husbands, husbands asking their elder brothers, elder brothers asking their clan leaders, and sometimes clan leaders telephoning more important leaders in other parts of the country. Often, permission was ultimately refused. There was no such thing as "following doctors' orders." The protocols and ritualized behaviors that have come to be expected in Western doctor–patient relationships were almost entirely absent in the Hmong doctor–patient situations. (Following the publication of Fadiman's book, the California hospital where Baby Lia was treated has now developed a 7-week training program designed to strengthen the trust between doctors and the Hmong shamans and community [Brown, 2009]).

Anthropologist Turner (1988) has suggested that rituals are the performance of a complex sequence of symbolic acts and efforts to manage social dramas or personal crises. We have had examples of both above: (a) the scene with the nurse and the surgeon surely illustrates a social drama composed of a complex sequence of symbolic acts, as does the story of the daughter caring for her mother; and (b) the Hmong story illustrates a situation of potential personal crisis. Turner's use of the word *performance* suggests again that rituals contain formalized roles and actions. The symbolization process is a tool of meaning (Fine, 1999); rituals are powerful contributors of meaning in our lives.

## DISABILITY AS DIFFERENCE

In occupational therapy, we often work with people who have disabilities. Within a cultural framework, people with disabilities represent a strongly ingrained "other" in many societies. The meaning of disability in a society is the amalgamation of people's definitions of difference compared to similarity. As Frank (2000) has stated, "disability is an artifact of culture," and further, "Disability is arbitrarily constructed and imposed on people, relegating them to a lower status and sometimes to an inescapable caste" (p. 168). Frank's words reflect the truism that the difference represented by disability in Western culture is almost inevitably an *undesirable* difference or, as Estroff called it, a "negative differentness" (Estroff, 1981, p. 220). Disability is a difference that stands in opposition to the "normative ideologies of the body" (Porter, 1997, p. xiv). Not until as recently as 1988 did somebody in the disabilities rights movement finally ask the question, "Can disability be beautiful?" (Hahn, 1988).

Attention to disability in Western society has been dominated by the biological, social, and cognitive sciences (Mitchell & Snyder, 1997). Defined as the presence of "cognitive and physical conditions that deviate from normative ideas of mental ability and physiological function" (p. 2), disabilities have long been regarded almost exclusively as debilitating phenomena that need medical intervention. In recent years, disability is being increasingly recognized as essentially a social experience in people's lives. The 1990 Americans With Disabilities Act offers support for this expanded social view of disability, as does the World Health Organization in its recently revised *International Classification of Disability*. The former includes stigma in its definition of disability, validating the importance of culture and social experience in the disability phenomenon. The latter includes limitations of participation in society as one of the major impacts of disability.

But the decades of focus on the body and its "impairments" of the past century continue to exert a major influence on our views of disability today. Those of us in the health professions are particularly vulnerable to its influence because one could say that we are, after all, dependent on this focus for our livelihood. If we are brave enough to step outside our world of rehabilitation and health care, we find examples of very harsh criticism indeed, aimed at what may be described as the self-serving nature of what we do. Mitchell and Snyder (1997), champions of this view from outside the health care arena, made the following statement:

> Historically, disability has been the province of numerous professional and academic disciplines that concentrate upon the management, repair, and maintenance of physical and cognitive incapacity. ... Medicine, rehabilitation, special education, sociology, psychology, and a panoply of subspecialties have all established their scientific and social credentials (as well as their very professional legitimacy) through the "humane" study and provision of services to disabled populations. ... We rarely consider that the continual circulation of professionally sponsored stories about disabled people's limitations, dependencies, and abnormalities proves necessary to the continuing existence of these professional fields of study. (p. 1)

I find it painful to read such characterizations of the work that we do. But part of the reason that it is painful is because statements such as these strike a chord deep within us that rings true. We *do* owe our existence and legitimacy to the fact that we, as health professionals, have strongly defined disability as the other, as different. We would not exist except that people, by virtue of the very fact that we define them as others, are in need of our services. In the rehabilitation framework, the assumption is made that people with disabilities need us to enable them to overcome the difference, or to at least be *less* different. To our way of thinking, we are enabling people to feel a sense of greater belonging within their families, communities, and the world through our treatment regimens. But writers such as Mitchell and Snyder (1997) are asking us to back up and look at ourselves as the creators of the need for the services that we provide, because we are also, like it or not, major contributors to the social forces that structure the otherness of disability.

## A Breach in Realities

For the masses of human beings in the world who fit the normative ideologies for physical and mental capabilities, people who present with disabilities interject what Estroff (1981) referred to as a "breach" into our realities. Because of this breach, the *differences* between us are what rule the relationship. In our culture, the disabled body "disturbs our deepest fascinations with the body, our fantasies of the body … the intrusion of a disabled body into these fantasies is disquieting in the extreme" (Porter, 1997, p. xiii. I use the word *body* here to include not only the corporeal body but also the mind and spirit.)

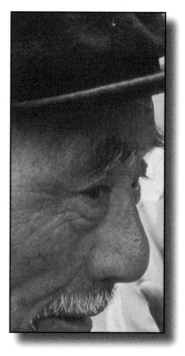

Davis (1997) used the term *abled gaze* (p. 52) to refer to the culturally determined perspective that people without disabilities have of those with disabilities in our society. He describes a social encounter with disability as "a disruption in the visual, auditory, or perceptual field" (p. 53), a description that is remarkably similar to Estroff's (1981) concept of the breach. The abled gaze is a gaze of power. The person who is gazing puts him- or herself in the position of the norm, the criterion against which others are compared, thus perpetuating and ever strengthening the social categories of abled and disabled and the division of the social world into normal and different. In this way, an encounter with disability is unbalanced because the "normal" person in the encounter has a repertoire of ableist assumptions and expectations that empower the gaze and the interaction.

In Gelya Frank's (2000) historiography of Diane DeVries, a woman born without arms or legs, Frank sought mightily to overcome the breach between herself and Diane and to understand the abled gaze, both aspects of her encounter with disability. Using what she called the "mirror phenomenon" (p. 4), Frank began her research by examining her own emotional responses to Diane, using reflection and introspection about her own life and experiences with disability: "First, I tried to remember all the people I knew who were 'crips' and my feelings about them. … Next I examined the ways in which, on the basis of physical limitations, *I* could be considered a 'crip' … Finally, because I perceived Diane's body as *missing* something, I examined experiences of lack and loss in my life" (p. 87). Through this process of self-reflection and examination of emotions, Frank came gradually to see Diane as a survivor, not a victim, and to focus on what was *right* with Diane, rather than on what was missing. The result of all this emotional and intellectual effort by the author was to successfully narrow the breach of realities that initially existed between herself and Diane DeVries and to moderate the power of the abled gaze. The imbalance of the encounter was lessened; the locus of power and decision making in their relationship was negotiated and renegotiated over the years as they sought to understand and reconcile their individual perspectives on the nature of their very strong affiliation with each other.

## The Paradox of Rehabilitation

I have stated that people in the health fields set goals and plan treatment in an effort to minimize each disabled person's differentness and to maximize each one's ability to share in the world of people who are able-bodied. The historian Stiker (1999) referred to the rehabilitation movement of the 20th century as an act of "un-difference" (p. 150), meaning that the overall goal of rehabilitation is to make everyone identical (i.e., to erase the differences). He called rehabilitation a "passport" for admission to be "like the others" (p. 151). "The face of society should not have any pimples," (p. 150) is Stiker's interpretation of the motivation behind rehabilitation; we should get rid of all the differences, thereby eliminating the breach and social disruption of ability/disability encounters.

Yet, in the view of many like others cited above, the nature of our work perpetuates the concept of disability by focusing on and legitimizing difference in the people for whom we provide services. In the United States, diagnostic labels are often required for access to our services; the nature of our treatment goals paradoxically calls attention to and promulgates the view of people with disabilities as being different, even though the stated aims are to lessen the differences and to increase the sense of participating membership in society. People must be categorized as different in order to be eligible to receive the services we offer to help them to be undifferent—to enable them to be like everyone else. Surely, we can all see what Stiker (1999) called the "flagrant" contradictions in this system of beliefs and services.

## *The Paradox of Disability*

People with disabilities are caught in the same paradox. Participants in Lupton and Seymour's study (2000) on selfhood and disability stated that they, on the one hand, appreciated the ways that many new technologies had enabled them to overcome aspects of their disabilities, but they also said that these same technologies served to mark them as "different." It's sort of a "damned if you do and damned if you don't" kind of situation. People with disabilities are caught between the need to recognize and accept their disabilities as part of themselves, and their desire to see themselves as "normal."

Goffman (1963) described how the person with a disability oscillates between identifying with the disabled community and identifying with the nondisabled community, experiencing what he called "affiliation cycles" (p. 38). The cycling represents the vacillations of the individual between acceptance of the special services and/or opportunities afforded to him or her because of the disabilities (e.g., funding for new assistive technologies) and a desire to reject the special services and, instead, to "pass" as normal. Or, as Estroff (1981) described in her study of people with mental illness, "clients not only accept and elaborate their differentness but also hate, fear, and reject it at the same time" (p. 235). Frank (2000) described Diane's experiences as a "crossing over, back and forth," between a common humanity and the distinctiveness of difference (p. 169). These words are all remarkably similar to each other—oscillations, vacillations, crossings, and affiliation cycles—and describe the lifelong paradox of living with a disability.

Stiker (1999) offered hope of a new outlook on disability, one that breaks out of the framework of sameness and difference.

> Let us stop seeing the able and disabled as normalcy and aberration, and let
> us no longer set them out as two separate kinds. ... We will not demand of

the disabled person that she [sic] resemble an able person. We will not make a person who is disabled into someone inherently disabled, more or less below the normal... the relationship between sound and less sound will always be treated relatively, dynamically, differently. This is the direction of future thought. (p. 194)

Stiker's thoughts are a sharp contrast to the widespread assumption that people with disabilities need to be changed, that they need rehabilitation.

If we are to begin to realize Stiker's (1999) hope for the future, we will need to moderate our tendency to divide the world into those who are able and those who are disabled; the relationship between sound and less sound will need to be treated relatively, dynamically. In this future world, we will be able to see the world as a many-peopled place, one full of all *kinds* of folks possessing a great variety of bodies and minds, all of which are "normal" in their own way relative to each other.

# REFERENCES

Agar, M. (1994). *Language shock: Understanding the culture of conversation.* New York, NY: William Morrow and Company.

American Occupational Therapy Association. (2008). Occupational therapy practice framework: Domain & process (2nd ed.). *American Journal of Occupational Therapy, 62,* 625-683.

Black, R., & Wells, S. (2007). *Culture and occupation: A model of empowerment in occupational therapy.* Bethesda, MD: AOTA Press.

Bonder, B., Martin, L., & Miracle, A. W. (2004). Culture emergent in occupation. *American Journal of Occupational Therapy, 58,* 159-168.

Brown, P. L. (2009, September 20). A doctor for disease, a shaman for the soul. *New York Times.*

Clark, F. A. (2000). The concepts of habit and routine: A preliminary theoretical synthesis. *Occupational Therapy Journal of Research, 20*(Suppl.), 123S-137S.

Crepeau, E. B. (1994). Three images of interdisciplinary team meetings. *American Journal of Occupational Therapy, 48,* 717-722.

Crepeau, E. B. (1995). Rituals. In C. B. Royeen (Ed.), *The practice of the future: Putting occupation back into therapy: Module 6.* Bethesda, MD: American Occupational Therapy Association.

Davis, L. (1997). Nude Venuses, Medusa's body, and phantom limbs: Disability and visuality. In D. T. Mitchell & S. L. Snyder (Eds.), *The body and physical difference: Discourses of disability* (pp. 51-70). Ann Arbor, MI: University of Michigan Press.

Dean, R. G. (2001). The myth of cross-cultural competence. *Families in Society: The Journal of Contemporary Human Services, 82,* 623-630.

Dewey, J. (1957). *Human nature and conduct: An introduction to social psychology.* New York, NY: Modern Library.

DiGiacomo, S. M. (1999). Can there be a "cultural epidemiology"? *Medical Anthropology Quarterly, 13,* 436-457.

Dillard, A. (1989). *The writing life.* New York, NY: Harper & Row.

Estroff, S. (1981). *Making it crazy: An ethnography of psychiatric clients in an American community.* Berkeley, CA: University of California Press.

Fadiman, A. (1997). *The spirit catches you and you fall down.* New York, NY: Farrar, Straus and Giroux.

Ferguson, M. (1980). *The aquarian conspiracy: Personal and social transformation in the 1980s.* Los Angeles, CA: J. P. Tarcher.

Fine, S. B. (1999). Symbolization: Making meaning for self and society. In G. Fidler & B. Velde (Eds.), *Activities: Reality and symbol* (pp. 11-25). Thorofare, NJ: SLACK Incorporated.

Fitzgerald, M. H. (2000). Establishing cultural competency for mental health professionals. In V. Skultans & J. Cox (Eds.), *Anthropological approaches to psychological medicine: Crossing bridges* (pp. 184-200). Philadelphia, PA: Jessica Kingsley.

Frank, G. (2000). *Venus on wheels: Two decades of dialogue on disability, biography, and being female in America.* Berkeley, CA: University of California Press.

Gallimore, R., & Lopez, E. M. (2002). Everyday routines, human agency, and ecocultural context: Construction and maintenance of individual habits. *OTJR: Occupation, Participation and Health, 22*(Suppl.), 70S-77S.

Geertz, C. (1973). *The interpretation of cultures: Selected essays.* New York, NY: Basic Books.

Goff, N. (2001, March). Outside looking in. *Wisconsin State Journal,* pp. 1-2.

Goffman, E. (1956). *The presentation of self in everyday life.* Edinburgh, UK: University of Edinburgh.

Goffman, E. (1963). *Stigma: Notes on the management of spoiled identity.* Englewood Cliffs, NJ: Prentice-Hall.

Gubrium, J. F., & Holstein, J. A. (2000). Introduction. In J. F. Gubrium & J. A. Holstein (Eds.) *Aging and everyday life* (pp. 1-11). Malden, MA: Blackwell Publishers.

Hahn, H. (1988). Can disability be beautiful? *Social Policy, 18,* 26-32.

Hammell, K. W. (2004). Dimensions of meaning in the occupations of daily life. *Canadian Journal of Occupational Therapy, 71,* 296-305.

Hammell, K. W. (2009). Sacred texts: A skeptical exploration of the assumptions underpinning theories of occupation. *Canadian Journal of Occupational Therapy, 76,* 6-13.

Illich, I. (1970). *Deschooling society.* Evanston, IL: Harper & Row.

Iwama, M. (2005). Situated meaning: An issue of culture, inclusion, and occupational therapy. In F. Kronenberg, S. S. Algado, & N. Pollard (Eds.), *Occupational therapy without borders* (pp. 127-139). New York, NY: Elsevier

Iwama, M. (2007). Culture and occupational therapy: Meeting the challenge of relevance in a global world. *Occupational Therapy International, 14,* 183-187.

Jungersen, K. (2002). Cultural safety: Kawa Whakaruruhau—An occupational therapy perspective. *New Zealand Journal of Occupational Therapy, 49,* 4-9.

Kalekin-Fishman, D. (1987). Performances and accounts: The social construction of the kindergarten experience. *Sociological Studies of Child Development, 2,* 81-104.

Krefting, L. H., & Krefting, D. V. (1991). Cultural influences on performance. In C. Christiansen & C. Baum (Eds.), *Occupational therapy: Overcoming human performance deficits* (pp. 100-122). Thorofare, NJ: SLACK Incorporated.

Lupton, D., & Seymour, W. (2000). Technology, selfhood and physical disability. *Social Science & Medicine, 50,* 1851-1862.

Malinowski, B. (1992). *Magic, science and religion.* Prospect Heights, IL: Waverland Press.

Mattingly, C., & Beer, D. W. (1993). Interpreting culture in a therapeutic context. In H. Hopkins & H. D. Smith (Eds.), *Willard and Spackman's occupational therapy* (8th ed., pp. 154-161). Philadelphia, PA: J. B. Lippincott & Co.

Mitchell, D. T., & Snyder, S. L. (1997). Introduction: Disability studies and the double bind of representation. In D. T. Mitchell & S. L. Snyder (Eds.), *The body and physical difference: Discourses of disability* (pp. 1 -31). Ann Arbor, MI: University of Michigan Press.

Myerhoff, B. (1977). We don't wrap herring in a printed page: Fusion, fictions, and continuity in secular ritual. In S. F. Moore & B. Myerhoff (Eds.), *Secular ritual* (pp. 199-223). Amsterdam, The Netherlands: Van Gorcum.

Odawara, E. (2005). Cultural competency in occupational therapy: Beyond a cross-cultural view of practice. *American Journal of Occupational Therapy, 59,* 325-334.

Ortner, S. B. (2006). *Anthropology and social theory: Culture, power, and the acting subject.* Durham, NC: Duke University Press.

Pollio, H. R., Henley, T., & Thompson, C. B. (1997). *The phenomenology of everyday life.* Cambridge, UK: Cambridge University Press.

Porter, J. I. (1997). Foreword. In D. T. Mitchell & S. L. Snyder (Eds.), *The body and physical difference: Discourses of disability* (p. xiii-xiv). Ann Arbor, MI: University of Michigan Press.

Rapoport, A. (1980). Cross-cultural aspects of environmental design. In I. Altman, A. Rapoport, & J. F. Wohlwill (Eds.), *Human behavior and environment* (Vol. 4, pp. 7-46). New York, NY: Plenum Press.

Stiker, H. J. (1999). *A history of disability.* Ann Arbor, MI: University of Michigan Press.

Tuan, Y. F. (1994). The city and human speech. *The Geographical Review, 84,* 144-151.

Turner, V. (1988). *The anthropology of performance.* New York, NY: PAJ Publications.

Whiteford, G. E., & Wilcock, A. A. (2000). Cultural relativism: Occupation and independence reconsidered. *Canadian Journal of Occupational Therapy, 67,* 324-336.

Wilcock, A. A. (1998). *An occupational perspective of health.* Thorofare, NJ: SLACK Incorporated.

Wilcock, A. A. (2006). *An occupational perspective of health* (2nd ed.). Thorofare, NJ: SLACK Incorporated.

Wolff, B. (2001, March). "Undesirable elements" reveals truths in cultural differences. *Wisconsin Week,* p. 9.

# OCCUPATION AS A
# SOURCE OF WELL-BEING
# AND DEVELOPMENT

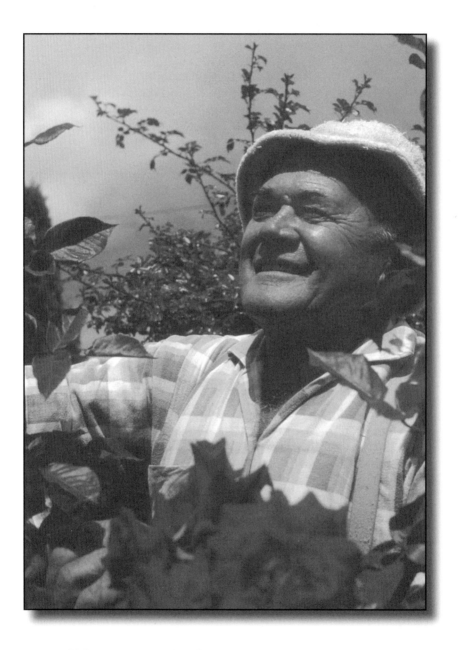

I would have a man to be doing, and to prolong his lives offices as much as lieth in him, and let death seize upon me whilest I am setting my cabiges, carelesse of her dart, but more of my unperfect garden.

*Montaigne* (in Mendel, 1939, p. 33)

Born in France in the year 1533, Montaigne authored a single book—the *Essays*. This lone, small book contains a collection of short writings that focus in an almost playful manner on the subject of self-knowledge. In the introduction to the publication cited above, Gide wrote of Montaigne, "… all other knowledge seemed to him uncertain; but the human being he discovers—and uncovers—is so genuine, so true, that in him every reader of the *Essays* recognizes himself" (p. 3). The book was enormously successful in its time, and its eclectic, flowing disclosures of Montaigne's self ("Everything in himself is an object of curiosity, amusement, and astonishment. …" p. 7) are as revealing today of the inner selves of ordinary people as they were of the people in the 16th century.

Montaigne's thoughts, quoted above, are from his essay, *Reflections on Death*. In these lines, Montaigne gives voice to the meaning life holds for him and to his hopes for the manner in which his life will end. He would have a person to be "doing" and able to continue that doing for as long as possible ("as much as lieth in him"). He hopes that his own death will come in the midst of his usual, everyday activity. Using the homely metaphor of his vegetable garden, Montaigne cries, "Let death seize upon me whilest I am setting my cabiges."

To me, this 16th-century passage expresses the essence of the meaning of occupation and the philosophy of occupational therapy. Engagement in life is the crux of meaning in life. To be able to "do" in daily life, and to be able to focus on the doing rather than on encroachments such as failing health—to Montaigne, this is the essence of how he wants to live his life. To use more modern language, this is the essence of well-being and lifelong development.

# THE ESSENCE OF WELL-BEING

Research on the human state of well-being is permeated by the belief that a person's ability to engage in life's daily activities is a key ingredient. This belief in the centrality of occupation to well-being is, perhaps obviously, strongly represented within our own profession and occupational therapy literature. Wood (1998), in her creative presentation of Occupatio as the allegorical representation of the occupational force in our lives, referred to this allegorical force as "life itself: that ubiquitous stream of transactions between humans and their worlds that is organized around recognizable activities *from which* whole constellations of skills and routines, identities and lifetimes, radiate" (p. 321). One cannot get much more fundamental than "life itself" in terms of identifying elements of well-being.

Wood (1998) described occupation as the central germinating force of life, with all else radiating out from that central force like spokes from the hub of a wheel. From this perspective, life without occupation would be tenuous and the experience of well-being would be nigh unto impossible. What meanings have others given to the term *well-being*?

Hasselkus, B. R.
*The Meaning of Everyday Occupation, Second Edition* (pp. 85-100).
© 2011 SLACK Incorporated

## The Good Life

Yi-Fu Tuan, humanistic geographer, published a book in 1986 with the title, *The Good Life*. To speak of the good life is to speak of well-being. Tuan set out in his book to understand the nature of the good life in modern society. According to Tuan, the good life includes elements of the *physical setting* in which we find ourselves, the *activities* in which we participate, our *philosophical understandings* of human nature and its virtues, and the *social harmony* we hope to bring about as we seek to realize Utopia. To Tuan, "The good life haunts us. Everything we do is directed, consciously or subconsciously, toward attaining it" (p. 6).

In Tuan (1986), then, we have a view of the good life or well-being that expands beyond Wood's occupational conceptualization. To be sure, Tuan named *activity* as one of four key elements of the good life, but he also specifically named our physical environments, our philosophical musings, and the social relationships we strive to perfect. Although we might incorporate some of Tuan's added dimensions into our concept of occupation (e.g., social interactions can be included as a form of occupation), I think we must recognize that his inclusion of the sort of cosmic dimensions of life—philosophical understandings and social harmony—expands our thinking of well-being beyond the realm of occupation per se.

## Positive Human Health

Ryff and Singer (1996, 1998) also spoke of the good life but from a psychological perspective. In their work published in 1996, Ryff and Singer described six key dimen-

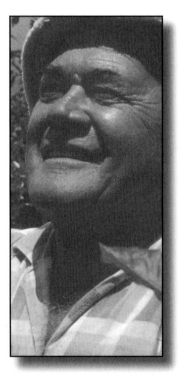

sions of well-being, based on a meta-analysis of theoretical literature on positive psychological functioning, lifespan development, and positive criteria for mental health. The six dimensions are self-acceptance, positive relations with others, autonomy, environmental mastery, purpose in life, and personal growth. They stated that there are "notable parallels between the formulations of wellness emerging from the literature and philosophical perspectives on the meaning of 'the good life'" (p. 16).

Ryff and Singer further developed their thesis in the work published in 1998 in which they offered a treatise on "positive human health." Determined to move beyond the medical model of health as the elimination of disease ("beyond repair shops," p. 1), Ryff and Singer defined well-being by two core features: (a) leading a life of purpose, and (b) quality connections to others. They summarized by saying, "positive health is ultimately about engagement in living" (p. 10). Thus, in the realm of psychological research on well-being, similar to Tuan's (1986) conceptualization of the good life, we again find purpose, engagement, and harmony in relations with others present as key dimensions.

Critiques of Ryff and Singer's (1998) treatise on positive human health have pointed to the absence of subjective well-being in their formulation of health (Diener, Sapyta, & Suh, 1998), the question about whether or not the characteristics listed are universally positive in all cultures and in all life circumstances (Diener et al.), and the oversimplification represented by the positive-negative distinction of health (Contrada, 1998; e.g., the failure to address life engagement that may represent both positive and negative factors such as the life of purpose embedded in belonging to a street gang). In regard to this last point, Ryff and Singer more recently modified their stance, calling for more nuanced distinctions that do not separate the human condition into positive and negative features (2003). In another critique, Spiegel (1998) put the *disease* back into the formulation for health, citing his experience with a support group for women with cancer who, despite the "negative" nature of their health, continued to have experiences of pleasure, happiness, and enjoyment in their lives. One woman's description of her long-awaited evening out at the Santa Fe Opera reflected her ability to have a gala evening, in spite of the presence of her disease: "I brought my cancer with me and put it in the seat next to me. It was there, but I had a wonderful time." Spiegel went on to say that, "Thinking of happiness as the absence of sadness is just as mistaken a notion as defining positive human health as the absence of disease. ... Thus, although good health is more than the absence of disease, disease does not imply the absence of happiness" (p. 67).

The conversation in psychology about the nature of well-being in life continues. Grappling with questions regarding the essential meaning of health, cultural universals of health, the relationship of happiness to positive health, the relationship of positive health to traditional medical care, the negative aspects of positive health and vice versa, and the meaning of health as distinct from its determinants emerges as the continuing research trajectory.

## Active Living

The interconnectedness between engagement in life and well-being is espoused in many other fields as well, such as public health, sports psychology, medical sociology, and gerontology. In their review of research and theory on relationships between activity and health, Frankish, Milligan, and Reid (1998) used the term *active living* to capture the essential meaning of a person's healthful engagement in life. Active living is a phrase that originated in Canada in the early 1990s (Active Living Canada, 1994; Health and Welfare Canada, 1991). The concept of active living represents a shift away from the view of fitness and activity as prescriptive, expert-guided, routinized pursuits. Instead, active living represents participation of the whole person—body, mind, and spirit—in a dynamic life, the meaning of which is relative to each person. Frankish et al. (1998) suggest that the concept of active living has historically been overly individualistic, focusing almost exclusively on the individual without a balance of emphasis on lifestyle features within their social and environmental contexts (strikingly similar to the concerns about occupational therapy referred to in chapter 2; Dickie, Cutchin, & Humphry, 2006; Hammell, 2009). To rectify this overemphasis on the individual, Frankish et al. proposed "the need to link the historically, individual-focused literature on physical activity/active living with the emerging recognition that sociocultural and structural determinants play a key role in influencing a wide range of activities of daily life" (p. 287).

The concept of active living, in both its individualistic and its broad sociocultural sense, fits well with Tuan's (1986) concept of the good life and with Ryff and Singer's (1996, 1998) concept of positive human health. Unlike Tuan or Ryff and Singer, however, Frankish et al. (1998) conceptualized active living within the framework of *determinants* of health. In Frankish et al., certain positive living conditions in life (such as wealth, education, age, social support) enhance the possibilities for active living and, in turn, active living enhances the potential for positive changes in living conditions and determinants of health. This reciprocal relationship is clearly evident in the study by Blakeney and Marshall (2009) on water quality, health, and occupation in a coal mining area of Kentucky. The authors stated in their results that "almost every daily occupation ... was affected by polluted water in the physical environment (watershed), as well as inside the home from well water or the municipal water supply" (p. 51). Whereas Tuan's good life and Ryff and Singer's contours of human health are described as *amalgams* of various dimensions of life that, when they occur together in certain ways, constitute well-being, Frankish et al. and Blakeney and Marshall are striving to identify *determinants* of well-being; sociocultural phenomena and conditions of community living are determinants they have identified.

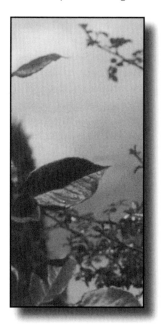

The circularity of mutual health benefits fostered by the interactions between active living and living conditions can be illustrated by an occupational therapist's story of a 16-year-old adolescent boy who sustained a spinal cord injury in a diving accident. According to the therapist, the teenager came to the rehabilitation center "really devastated by the accident because he was very active, very athletic, very outgoing. ..."

> With the use of EMG biofeedback and everything else we were doing in therapy, just general ADLs and strengthening activities and isolated muscle strengthening ... he's regained a lot of function in his hands, his arms; he's got a car now, he's independent in transfers back and forth from the car. He had a job this summer at the pool. He's just really—he was really depressed when he first came and has really turned around, he's come a long way. And he's also up walking a little bit now in physical therapy, with a walker, and just doing a lot of really wonderful things. I've seen a real change in his attitude, too. He's back in the social swing of things and just really has come a long, long, long way. And we're still working; he's still making progress.

In this scenario, we see the resources of the health care system, likely coupled with other resources such as family, economic security, friendships, inner drive, etc., enhancing the potential for active living in this 16-year-old adolescent. Reciprocally, the evolving participation of the youth in active living facilitates "a change in his attitude" and reinvolvement in life's activities. "He had a job this summer at the pool," and "he's back in the social swing of things," illustrate not only individual achievements such as increased strength and the ability to drive his car but also changes within the boy's sociocultural environment; that is, within the social world of adolescents in Western culture. The health-promoting circularity of active living has been realized. Life is returning to a pattern of "engagement in living" (Ryff & Singer, 1998, p. 10), and the ingredients of Tuan's (1986) good life are reappearing, specifically activity, a supportive physical environment, harmony in relations with others, and a positive personal philosophy of life.

## A Sense of Coherence

Another sociologist, Aaron Antonovsky, and his colleagues (1993; Antonovsky & Sagy, 1986; Antonovsky & Sourani, 1988) extend our thinking further about the positive conditions or resources of life that enhance our potential for enjoying health and well-being. Again, partly in reaction to the pathogenic orientation (the "repair shops") that for so long dominated Western conceptions of health, Antonovsky (1993) focused instead on the resources of life, such as education and cultural stability, seeking to uncover whatever it was about these resources that enabled them to promote health. The theoretical concept that evolved from Antonovsky's thinking was the *sense of coherence*: "Resources were seen as leading to life experiences which promoted the development of a strong SOC [sense of coherence], a way of seeing the world which facilitated successful coping with the innumerable, complex stressors confronting us in the course of living" (p. 725).

According to Antonovsky (1993), to possess a sense of coherence is to perceive one's world as comprehensible, manageable, and meaningful. In such a world, the internal and external stimuli of a person's daily living are predictable and understandable, the resources needed to meet the demands posed by these stimuli are available, and the demands of these stimuli are valued—they matter.

The "manageability" component of Antonovsky's (1993) sense of coherence is especially compelling to me. When I was working on my doctoral degree, Antonovsky's theoretical model of coherence was not yet fully developed, and I was not aware of him or the emerging model. My dissertation was an ethnographic study of family caregiving for elderly in the community (Hasselkus, 1988, 1989). The data were more than 800 pages of text from 60 taped interviews with 15 family caregivers, focusing on their daily activities and routines of caring for elderly relatives. I generated six interpretive themes of meaning from the data (Hasselkus, 1988); the theme that seemed the most ethnographic to me was *a sense of managing*. Within a sense of managing, family members talked about wanting to have things "pretty well under control," wanting to be able to "get things done," being able to maintain personal standards of orderliness and cleanliness, and keeping the costs of caregiving down to an affordable level. In occupational therapy terms, manageability for the caregivers meant being able to balance the occupational demands of the day and feeling up to the challenges that came along.

In my study, one family caregiver had been instructed by a therapist to put sandbags on her husband's leg "every hour," leaving her wondering how "I would ever get my work done." As it turned out, this caregiver devised a way to be able to get her work done *and* attend to her husband's leg; on her own, she started a daily exercise routine for her husband that she carried out each morning while he was still in bed:

> I just kinda started doing this on my own so I'd know he could get it straightened out. So I'd just bend it [the leg] up and help him get it straightened out, and bend it up and keep doing that and then hold it down straight on the bed for a while … it seems to work pretty well—I got his leg so it straightens out real good.

With this modification in her daily occupations, life for this caregiver was once again comprehensible, manageable, and meaningful; she was able to reconcile the conflicting demands of two valued activities (i.e., her work and the caregiving). In Antonovsky's terms, a sense of coherence had been reestablished.

## Synthesis Through Occupation

The good life, positive human health, active living, and a sense of coherence are four representations of well-being in modern Western life. The findings of a small qualitative study on the meaning of health to a sample of occupational therapists in Sweden are remarkably similar to these grander theories (Björklund & Svensson, 2000). The meanings of health generated by this Swedish sample of therapists were collapsed during the analysis into three primary themes: health as feeling fine, health as the ability to act, and health as an objective state of the body and/or the mind. Canadians Rebeiro and Cook (1999) offered another term to synthesize the health-promoting power of occupation—"occupational spin-off" (p. 176). Occupational spin-off contains health-sustaining aspects of life such as affirmation of self and confirmation of accomplishments.

Perhaps the best synthesis to date of these considerations within an occupational therapy framework is what has become known as the well-elderly study carried out at the University of Southern California in the mid-1990s (Clark et al., 1997; Jackson, Carlson, Mandel, Zemke, & Clark, 1998). In this randomized controlled trial study, three groups of multiethnic, well-elderly people in the community—an occupational therapy treatment group, a social activity control group, and a nontreatment control group—were compared on a number of outcome measures, including depression, life satisfaction, physical and social function, and self-rated health. The key intent of the 9 months of occupational therapy treatment was "to help the participants better appreciate the importance of meaningful activity in their lives, as well as to impart specific knowledge about how to select or perform activities so as to achieve a healthy and satisfying lifestyle" (Clark et al., p. 1322).

Statistically significant benefits attributable to the occupational therapy treatment were found on the measures of quality of social interaction, life satisfaction, health perceptions, and health status, including improvements on measures of pain, role limitations, physical functioning, vitality, social functioning, and general mental health. The researchers concluded that the benefits of the occupational therapy treatment could be attributed to three key aspects of the treatment: (a) the therapy program enabled the participants to construct daily routines that were health promoting and meaningful in the context of their own lives; (b) the occupational therapy was highly individualized (in contrast to the social activity control group); and (c) the program included specific

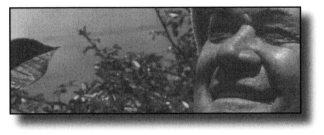

instruction on how to overcome barriers to successful daily living such as limited incomes and lack of awareness or knowledge about community support services.

Jackson et al. (1998) stated that the intent of the well-elderly program was "to enable each participant to determine which occupations affected his or her sense of well-being. Equipped with this knowledge, each participant was positioned to begin to thoughtfully weave his or her occupations into a coherent personalized health-promoting pattern" (p. 330). In the well-elderly study, we can readily see the ingredients of well-being: engagement in living, activity, meaningfulness, manageability, comprehensibility, strengthened resources, purpose, community involvement, and a supportive physical environment. The well-elderly study provides a compelling illustration of the power of occupation to enhance well-being in people's lives.

## Relative Well-Being

An alternative concept—*relative* well-being—has proven useful in describing situations in which people are experiencing certain aspects of active living and coherence in their lives, while also living with significant health problems and disharmony (Hasselkus, 1998; Perrin, 1997; Sandqvist, Äkesson, & Eklund, 2005). For example, Perrin used the terms *well-being/ill-being* and *minimal well-being* (p. 935) as well as *relative well-being* to capture the marginal and often fleeting moments of positive health experienced by people with severe dementia. In reference to the central role of occupation to the creation and existence of even these fleeting moments, Perrin stated, "Clearly, many staff do not have a problem sustaining interaction during a task-oriented activity such as feeding, bathing, or dressing. ... The difficulty of engagement with the severely impaired person arises when there are no more tasks left to be done" (p. 940). Relative well-being for the person with dementia may consist of a smile, eye contact, an attentive posture, laughter, or visual tracking—however momentary the behavior. In a study of women with cutaneous systemic sclerosis (Sandqvist et al.), relative well-being meant coexisting high satisfaction with social aspects of their lives (living situations, family relations) and low satisfaction with physical health. Authors in this study stated that the "vast majority of the women [in their study] with limited scleroderma were satisfied with their daily occupations and had a 'good life,' even though they were less satisfied than healthy women in certain aspects of daily occupations and well-being" (p. 395).

# OCCUPATION AND HUMAN DEVELOPMENT

On February 9, 2000, the late edition of *The New York Times* newspaper carried an article by Sara Rimer entitled, "Turning to Autobiography for Emotional Growth in Old

Age." Datelined Galveston, Texas, the article was about a writers' group that met twice-monthly in the backroom of a seafood restaurant, across Seawall Boulevard from the Gulf of Mexico. The people in the group ranged in age from their mid-60s to mid-80s. Said Rimer, "These new memoirists are writing for the same reasons writers have always written: to search for meaning in their lives, to find their voice, to leave a record. ... When done with a skilled guide and with sympathetic listeners, [the writing] can be a key to emotional growth in old age."

Linking writing to emotional growth in old age is one example of how occupation is linked to human development across the lifespan. In chapter 2, I introduced Wilcock's concept of becoming (1998); that is, the growth and transformation that is born of our engagement in living across the lifespan. Jackson et al. (1998) articulated the central tenet of occupational science as the belief that "humans are caught up in a world of occupations through which the self is continually constructed and disclosed. It is through one's immersion in the world of occupations that new discoveries about one's potential and a forward movement of one's life take place" (p. 329). Statements and concepts such as these lead us to the consideration of occupation within a lifespan context.

## The Lifespan Context for Occupation

The development of the human being across the lifespan has been variously characterized as a sequence of life passages (Sheehy, 1976, 1995), a life cycle of seasons (Levinson, 1978), a lifelong composition (Bateson, 1989), and a life narrative (Bruner, 1986; Mattingly, 1991, 1998). More recently, Iwama (2005) introduced an East Asian metaphor for lifespan development—the Kawa (river) model. In the Kawa model, "Life is a complex, profound journey that flows through time and space like a river"; further, the model encompasses "the perspective of harmony in life between self and context, and its relationship to well-being" (p. 218). The term *human development* has typically been used to refer to patterned sequences of changes in the human being that occur over a length of time (Kaluger & Kaluger, 1984). The metaphors used to characterize human development (a cycle of seasons, a composition, a river) are attempts to describe the patterns or rhythms of change that occur across the lifespan.

Much of our training and practice in occupational therapy reflects a lifespan developmental context. Therapists describe their practices as being "in pediatrics" or "in geriatrics," or therapists may consider themselves specialists in infant and neonatal care or adolescent care; the language used to describe these areas of practice is derived from a view of life as a sequence of phases. Occupational therapy curriculums throughout the world contain courses that are titled with these same terms.

In keeping with this developmental perspective, new areas of practice have arisen that focus on clients who are making life transitions, such as young people in the community shifting from years of foster care to independent adulthood (Paul-Ward, 2009) or older adults who are shifting into retirement (Jonsson, Josephsson, & Kielhofner, 2000). Grandmothers taking on care of new grandchildren, older folks who are giving up driving, mothers passing down recipes and holiday cooking traditions to daughters and grandchildren are other examples of life transitions being recognized, addressed in practice, and researched in occupational therapy (Ludwig, Hattjar, Russell, & Winston, 2007; Vrkljan & Polgar, 2007; Wright-St. Clair, Bunrayong, Vittayakorn, Rattakorn, & Hocking, 2004). Transitional therapy, by definition, reflects thinking about life as a series of shifts, sequences, and phases.

## Occupation as a Transformative Process

Belief in the ability to enhance lifelong human development through occupation is one of the core tenets of our profession. As Townsend has stated, "The active process of occupation ... enables humans to develop as individuals and as members of society" (1997, p. 19). Townsend referred to the developmental power of occupation as its transformative potential; "... this active process [of occupation] is the means for learning about the self and society, organizing life, discovering meaning, and exercising control" (p. 24).

In Townsend (1997), we find the extension of our earlier discussion of the writings of Palmer (2000) and Christiansen (1999); that is, Palmer's endorsement to "let your life speak" and Christiansen's declaration of the "selfing" that occurs through occupation. The theme of "becoming" through occupation occurs again and again in our literature (Fidler & Fidler, 1978; Kielhofner, 2008; Watson & Swartz, 2004; Wilcock, 1993, 2006), variously expressed as transformation, differentiation, development, and self-actualization. In her research, Urbanowski (2005) used the term *transformative processes* to refer to the personal development that accompanies life-changing events for both occupational therapists and clients in their work together (p. 302). Watson and Swartz used transformation in the title of their book about the power of occupation to change the lives of people in South Africa who live with violence, poverty, and discrimination on a day-to-day basis.

On another aspect of becoming, Unruh (2004) has written about the concept of occupational identity as a source of continuity across the lifespan. This concept was also borne out by women in a cross-cultural study of holiday cooking; "Talk about recipes and kitchen things used, and how the foods are prepared and served revealed layers of identity" (Wright-St. Clair, Hocking, Bunrayong, Vittayakorn, & Rattakorn, 2005, p. 332). Similarly, in a different context, engagement in familiar everyday occupations helped family caregivers "meet the challenges and live through the biographical disruption that accompanies the dementia caregiving experience" (Hasselkus & Murray, 2007, p. 12).

The embeddedness of occupation in lifespan human development may be the most powerful dimension of the relationship between occupation and well-being. As an essential element of developmental well-being, lifespan meaningful occupation appears to be an absolutely *universal* phenomenon—worldwide, across all cultures, among all people. Human beings thrive and develop through their occupational endeavors. It is impossible to envision lifespan development occurring without occupation. How eagerly we provide varieties of stimulation to foster the emerging physical and intellectual accomplishments of the developing infant and child, and how strongly those occupations symbolize for us the child's developmental progress. For people of all ages, the occupations of daily life can both foster development and provide visible signs of the development that is occurring. To understand the relationship of occupation and lifespan development better is a quintessential goal (perhaps even *the* quintessential goal) for occupational therapy researchers.

## Occupation as Lifelong Experience

In the book by Susan Gordon Lydon (1997) titled *The Knitting Sutra: Craft as a Spiritual Practice,* Lydon wrote eloquently about her passion for knitting and about the personal growth and development that the craft of knitting has brought her. "After all," she says, "the important thing is not so much what you knit as what happens to you while you knit it. Where the interior journey takes you. What you find there. How you are transformed when you come back home." Later in the book, Lydon stated further, "The purpose of the craft is not so much to make beautiful things as it is to become beautiful inside while you are making those things" (p. 137). It is the *experience* of the craft that moves one along in making life's journey. So, too, it is the experience of *all* occupation that moves one along in making life's journey.

This concept of the primacy of the experience of craft rather than the product is powerfully represented in the art of the Australian Aboriginal peoples (Morphy, 1998). In his scholarly and stunningly illustrated book, Morphy informed the reader, that, "Much Aboriginal art was (and is) indeed largely invisible and not collectible. It is frequently produced in the context of rituals, is often intended to be ephemeral and may even be deliberately destroyed during the course of the ceremony or allowed to disappear naturally within a few days of its completion" (p. 23). For example, body paintings and ground sculptures (literally areas of "ground" that are sculpted into symbolic shapes) are meant to last only a few hours. To the Aboriginal people, the act of producing the art is as important as, or *more* important than, the finished object. Once

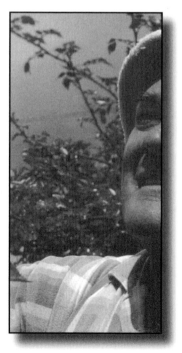

again, to paraphrase Lydon (1997), it is not so much what you create as what happens to you while you create it. It is the spirit of the *experience* of the occupation that moves one along life's journey.

In an interesting article in the April 2000 *Anthropology News*, cultural anthropologist Thomas Maschio lamented the American consumer culture that is so strongly manifested in the typically Western materialistic desire for goods and domestic products. According to Maschio, this desire for things has displaced life experience as "a way of becoming" (p. 7). Americans buy products as a way to create possibilities "about life, status, achievement, beauty, youth, athleticism, control, self-mastery, physical prowess, speed, safety, comfort, sex, intoxication, taste, food, scent, home, and love" (p. 7). The product is made into "an ally" in the contest to realize an idealized image of the self; further, the ownership of products becomes a vehicle for a feeling of well-being. Maschio presented the North American focus on products and things for meaning in life as the antithesis of the focus on *experience* that is present in many cultures.

In fact, Morphy (1998), in his book on Australian Aboriginal art, illustrated this tension between those who value the means and those who value the ends in his discussion of the differences between the views of the indigenous people and those of the European colonials who came to Australia in the late 1700s. At the time when Aboriginal art became recognized as *art*, the Western settlers grew interested in collecting and owning "pieces" of it. This desire for individual ownership of artistic works clashed with the Aboriginal concepts of art as an experience of connection to the ancestral beings, to the Dreamtime, to kinship ties, and to clanship and regional identity. To the Aboriginal peoples, the important meanings of the artwork lay in the execution of the art, much more than in the final product itself. Hence the frustration of potential collectors of Aboriginal art who saw desired artwork washed away by the rain or carved into the surface of a dead tree trunk!

The late writer Kurt Vonnegut (1999) also commented on the misplaced focus of Western peoples on things:

> ... people are being cheated out of the experience of "becoming." It's the computer which becomes now. People think, "Oh, boy, wait until I get this new program." Bill Gates will give you a program to write a perfect Shakespearean sonnet. For God's sake, that's not becoming. ... People should practice an art in order to *make their souls grow* [emphasis added] and not to make money or become famous. Paint a picture. Write.

In other words, according to Vonnegut, we should engage in occupation in order to "make our souls grow," to nourish our inner beings and promote our lifelong development. In Western society, because of our emphasis on material things and products, we often ignore the journey and focus instead on the destination. To Vonnegut and others, the journey itself is the crux of life; the accouterments along the way are but signposts for the journey.

## Phenomenological Occupation and the Person

To focus on the inner being and the transforming development of humans as they live their lives is to take a phenomenological view of the person and of occupation (Benner & Wrubel, 1989; Heidegger, 1962). In the phenomenological view, a person is a self-interpreting being; "the person does not come into the world predefined but becomes defined in the course of living a life" (Benner & Wrubel, p. 41). Further, the things and objects of the world are never separate from the person's *experience* of them (Breytspraak, 1984); only through a self that is experiencing the offerings of the world do our lives have coherence. As Pollio, Henley, and Thompson (1997) stated, "selfhood is always a becoming and is never complete in character" (p. 274).

The phenomenological view of the self is one of intimacy between a person's inner sense of experience and his or her encounters with the world. This view holds that, throughout our lives, because of the unceasing streams of experience that are present within our worlds, we *become*. Each instance of authentic experiencing in our daily lives demands anew from us consideration of what is possible for us. We are always balancing the actual with the possible. The changes that signify our lifespan transformation and development are the result of this dynamic balancing act, born of our lifelong efforts to let our lives speak at the same time that we reach toward the possible.

Examples of these lifelong transformative occupational encounters with the world are infinite in number for each one of us. Day after day, week after week, year after year, as we live out the ordinary and the dramatic aspects of our daily lives, we grow and develop through occupation. We consciously and subconsciously consider the balance in our lives and make choices about what occupations we will continue, which ones we will drop from our repertoire, and what possible new ventures we will take on.

Lo and behold, I was persuaded, at age 49, by a particularly skilled dental hygienist, to begin to floss my teeth daily, an occupation that, according to her, is directly linked to my well-being. In cultivating this new habit, I was, in effect, letting go of a previous bedtime ritual that did *not* include this task; as well, I was taking on a new occupation that took a small chunk of time out of my busy day and that forced upon me far greater intimacy with my teeth than I was accustomed to experiencing! In the larger scheme of life, my acceptance of this new daily responsibility signified exactly that—a shift from attributing responsibility for my oral hygiene to the dentist and the dental hygienist to attributing responsibility to myself for a larger proportion of this occupation. I, inexplicably, had weighed the balance between letting things be and trying something new and had made the choice to reach for new possibilities (however mundane this particular example might be). The change represented by this choice was reflected not only in my daily occupational routines but, in a small way, also in my way of being in the world.

And so it is with all the occupational events of our lives. The small stuff and the big stuff of life contribute to the development of each one of us across the lifespan. New ventures shift the balance of our days and new ventures shift the nature of our inner selves. Possibilities that are taken on inevitably result in accommodations in other aspects of our lives, as we continually seek to balance the actual with the possible. Whether it be learning a foreign language, joining a hand bell choir, writing a grant, seeing a patient who has a diagnosis that is unfamiliar, babysitting for a new granddaughter, taking that first trip to Europe, joining a writers' group, or *whatever* else one can think of—these are occupational endeavors about which we ponder as we consider the existing balance of our lives and the changes that will be brought about by the possibilities inherent in these new ventures.

Townsend (1997) has defined occupation as "the active process of everyday living" (p. 19). I would tend to speak of occupation as the *experience* of everyday living. Occupation acts as the vehicle by which people experience their worlds. As such, occupation is also the vehicle by which people encounter the possible, as individuals and as members of society, and through which lifespan change and development occur.

## OCCUPATION TO THE END

Law, Steinwender, and Leclair (1998) declared that available research evidence provides support for strong relationships between occupation and health and well-being.

Further, the influence of mediating factors, such as the perceived *experience* of the occupation, "enhances the effect of occupation on health" (p. 90). So we have occupation *and* the experience of occupation—both important to health and well-being, both contributing to the good life, to positive human health, to active living, and to coherence in life. Both are important across the lifespan, propelling us along the journeys of our lives as we strive daily to sort out and make choices about the actual and possible.

It seems appropriate to close this chapter with a final quote from Montaigne's *Essays*. This time, instead of using his vegetable garden, Montaigne aptly expresses his sentiments about life's ending using a metaphor taken from his lifelong experience of traveling the countryside on horseback. Translated into the charm of 16th-century English, Montaigne makes one more statement about his desire to remain active throughout his life: "I should chuse to weare out my life with my bum in the saddle, ever riding" (Mendel, 1939, p. 114). Enough said.

# REFERENCES

Active Living Canada. (1994). *Active living assembly summary report*. Ottawa, Ontario, Canada: Kent Consulting Ltd.

Antonovsky, A. (1993). The structure and properties of the sense of coherence scale. *Social Science & Medicine, 35,* 725-733.

Antonovsky, A., & Sagy, S. (1986). The development of a sense of coherence and its impact on responses to stress situations. *Journal of Social Psychology, 126,* 213-225.

Antonovsky, A., & Sourani, T. (1988). Family sense of coherence and family adaptation. *Journal of Marriage and the Family, 50,* 79-92.

Bateson, M. C. (1989). *Composing a life*. New York, NY: Plume.

Benner, P., & Wrubel, J. (1989). *The primacy of caring: Stress and coping in health and illness*. Menlo Park, CA: Addison-Wesley.

Björklund, A., & Svensson, T. (2000). Health, the body and occupational therapy. *Scandinavian Journal of Occupational Therapy, 7,* 26-32.

Blakeney, A. B., & Marshall, A. (2009). Water quality, health, and human occupations. *American Journal of Occupational Therapy, 63,* 46-57.

Breytspraak, L. M. (1984). *The development of self in later life*. Boston, MA: Little, Brown and Company.

Bruner, J. (1986). *Actual minds: Possible worlds*. Cambridge, MA: Harvard University Press.

Christiansen, C. (1999). Defining lives: Occupation as identity: An essay on competence, coherence, and the creation of meaning. *American Journal of Occupational Therapy, 53,* 547-558.

Clark, F., Azen, S. P., Zemke, R., Jackson, J., Carlson, M., Hay, J.,…Lipson, L. (1997). Occupational therapy for independent-living older adults. *Journal of the American Medical Association, 278,* 1321-1326.

Contrada, R. J. (1998). Commentary: It is easier to accentuate the positive in the absence of physical disease. *Psychological Inquiry, 9,* 29-33.

Dickie, V., Cutchin, M. P., & Humphry, R. (2006). Occupation as transactional experience: A critique of individualism in occupational science. *Journal of Occupational Science, 13,* 83-93.

Diener, E., Sapyta, J. J., & Suh, E. (1998). Commentary: Subjective well-being is essential to well-being. *Psychological Inquiry, 9*, 33-37.

Fidler, G. S., & Fidler, J. W. (1978). Doing and becoming: Purposeful action and self-actualization. *American Journal of Occupational Therapy, 32*, 305-310.

Frankish, C. J., Milligan, C. D., & Reid, C. (1998). A review of relationships between active living and determinants of health. *Social Science & Medicine, 47*, 287-301.

Hammell, K. W. (2009). Sacred texts: A skeptical exploration of the assumptions underpinning theories of occupation. *Canadian Journal of Occupational Therapy, 76*, 6-13.

Hasselkus, B. R. (1988). Meaning in family caregiving: Perspectives on caregiver/professional relationships. *The Gerontologist, 28*, 686-691.

Hasselkus, B. R. (1989). The meaning of daily activity in family caregiving for the elderly. *American Journal of Occupational Therapy, 43*, 649-656.

Hasselkus, B. R. (1998). Occupation and well-being in dementia: The experience of daycare staff. *American Journal of Occupational Therapy, 52*, 423-434.

Hasselkus, B. R., & Murray, B. J. (2007). Everyday occupation, well-being and identity: The experience of caregivers in families with dementia. *American Journal of Occupational Therapy, 61*, 9-20.

Health and Welfare Canada. (1991). *Active living: A conceptual overview*. Ottawa, Ontario, Canada: Author.

Heidegger, M. (1962). *Being and time* (Macquarrie & Robinson, Trans.). San Francisco, CA: Harper Collins.

Iwama, M. K. (2005). The Kawa (river) model: Nature, life flow, and the power of culturally relevant occupational therapy. In F. Kronenberg, S. Algado, & N. Pollard (Eds.), *Occupational therapy without borders* (pp. 213-227). New York, NY: Elsevier.

Jackson, J., Carlson, M., Mandel, D., Zemke, R., & Clark F. (1998). Occupation in lifestyle redesign: The Well Elderly Study Occupational Therapy Program. *American Journal of Occupational Therapy, 52*, 326-336.

Jonsson, H., Josephsson, S., & Kielhofner, G. (2000). Evolving narratives in the course of retirement: A longitudinal study. *American Journal of Occupational Therapy, 54*, 463-470.

Kaluger, G., & Kaluger, M. F. (1984). *Human development: The span of life*. St. Louis, MO: Times Mirror/Mosby.

Kielhofner, G. (2008). *Model of human occupation: Theory and application* (4th ed.). Baltimore, MD: Lippincott Williams & Wilkins.

Law, M., Steinwender, S., & Leclair, L. (1998). Occupation, health and well-being. *Canadian Journal of Occupational Therapy, 65*, 81-91.

Levinson, D. J. (1978). *The seasons of a man's life*. New York, NY: Alfred A. Knopf.

Ludwig, F. M., Hattjar, B., Russell, R. L., & Winston, K. (2007). How caregiving for grandchildren affects grandmothers' meaningful occupations. *Journal of Occupational Science, 14*, 40-51.

Lydon, S. G. (1997). *The knitting sutra: Craft as a spiritual practice*. San Francisco, CA: Harper Collins.

Maschio, T. (2000, April). The culture of desire. *Anthropology News*, 7-8.

Mattingly, C. (1991). The narrative nature of clinical reasoning. *American Journal of Occupational Therapy, 45*, 998-1005.

Mattingly, C. (1998). *Healing dramas and clinical plots: The narrative structure of experience*. Cambridge, UK: Cambridge University Press.

Mendel, A. O. (Ed.). (1939). *The living thoughts of Montaigne: Presented by Andre Gide*. Philadelphia, PA: David McKay Company.

Morphy, H. (1998). *Aboriginal art*. London, UK: Phaidon Press United.

Palmer, P. J. (2000). *Let your life speak: Listening for the voice of vocation*. San Francisco, CA: Jossey-Bass.

Paul-Ward, A. (2009). Social and occupational justice barriers in the transition from foster care to independent adulthood. *American Journal of Occupational Therapy, 63,* 81-88.

Perrin, T. (1997). Occupational need in severe dementia: A descriptive study. *Journal of Advanced Nursing, 25,* 934-941.

Pollio, H. R., Henley, T., & Thompson, C. B. (1997). *The phenomenology of everyday life*. Cambridge, UK: Cambridge University Press.

Rebeiro, K. L., & Cook, J. V. (1999). Opportunity, not prescription: An exploratory study of the experience of occupational engagement. *Canadian Journal of Occupational Therapy, 66,* 176-187.

Ryff, C. D., & Singer, B. (1996). Psychological well-being. Meaning, measurement and implications for psychotherapy research. *Psychotherapy & Psychosomatics, 65,* 14-23.

Ryff, C. D., & Singer, B. (1998). The contours of positive human health. *Psychological Inquiry, 9,* 1-28.

Ryff, C. D., & Singer, B. (2003). Ironies of the human condition: Well-being and health on the way to mortality. In L. G. Aspinwall & U. M. Straudinger (Eds.), *Fundamental questions and future directions for a positive psychology* (pp. 271-287). Washington, DC: American Psychological Association.

Sandqvist, G., Äkesson, A., & Eklund, M. (2005). Daily occupations and well-being in women with limited cutaneous systemic sclerosis. *American Journal of Occupational Therapy, 59,* 390-397.

Sheehy, G. (1976). *Passages: Predictable crises of adult life*. New York, NY: E. P. Dutton.

Sheehy, G. (1995). *New passages: Mapping your life across time*. New York, NY: Random House.

Spiegel, D. (1998). Getting there is half the fun: Relating happiness to health. *Psychological Inquiry, 9,* 66-68.

Townsend, E. (1997). Occupation: Potential for personal and social transformation. *Journal of Occupational Science: Australia, 4*(1), 18-26.

Tuan, Y. F. (1986). *The good life*. Madison, WI: University of Wisconsin Press.

Unruh, A. M. (2004). Reflections on: "So … what do you do?" Occupation and the construction of identity. *Canadian Journal of Occupational Therapy, 71,* 290-295.

Urbanowski, R. (2005). Transcending practice borders through perspective transformation. In F. Kronenberg, S. S. Algado, & N. Pollard (Eds.), *Occupational therapy without borders* (pp. 302-312). New York, NY: Elsevier.

Vonnegut, K. (1999, September 13). People. *Wisconsin State Journal*.

Vrkljan, B. H., & Polgar, J. M. (2007). Linking occupational participation and occupational identity: An exploratory study of the transition from driving to driving cessation in older adulthood. *Journal of Occupational Science, 14,* 30-39.

Watson, R., & Swartz, L. (2004). *Transformation through occupation*. London, UK: Whurr Pub.

Wilcock, A. A. (1993). A theory of the human need for occupation. *Journal of Occupational Science: Australia, 1,* 17-24.

Wilcock, A. A. (1998). *An occupational perspective of health*. Thorofare, NJ: SLACK Incorporated.

Wilcock, A. A. (2006). *An occupational perspective of health* (2nd ed.). Thorofare, NJ: SLACK Incorporated.

Wood, W. (1998). The genius within. *American Journal of Occupational Therapy, 52,* 320-325.

Wright-St. Clair, V., Bunrayong, W., Vittayakorn, S., Rattakorn, P., & Hocking, C. (2004). Offerings: Food traditions of older Thai women at Sonkran. *Journal of Occupational Science, 11,* 115-124.

Wright-St. Clair, V., Hocking, C., Bunrayong, W., Vittayakorn, S., & Rattakorn, P. (2005). Older New Zealand women doing the work of Christmas: A recipe for identity formation. *The Sociological Review, 53,* 332-350.

CHAPTER 6

# OCCUPATION AS MEANINGFUL CONNECTION

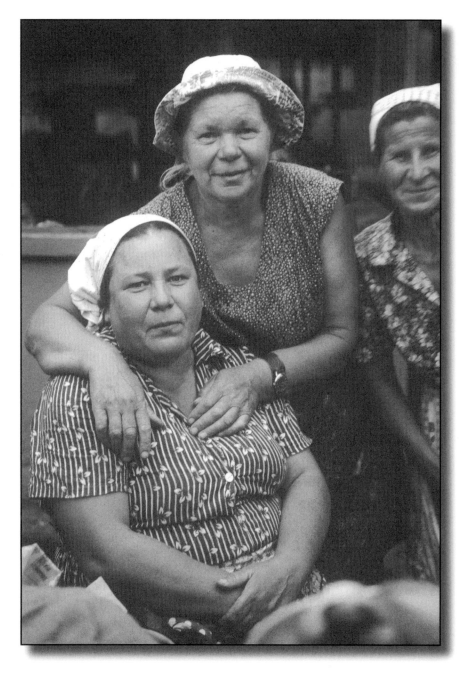

In the beginning is relation ...

Martin Buber (1958, p. 18)

"In the beginning is relation ..." says Martin Buber, a twentieth-century German philosopher, in his landmark book, *I and Thou* (1958). To Buber, relation (i.e., connectedness, being with) is the essential element of our existence in this world. We humans *dwell* in our relation; we are only truly present in the world as we exist *in relation* to other human beings, to nature, and the objects around us. "All real living is meeting" (p. 11). It is in and through relation, meeting, connection that our lives are authentically lived.

Relation and connection as core meanings of life is a concept expressed by others. Berger and Luckman (1966) echoed this theme from a sociological perspective: "I cannot exist in everyday life without continually interacting and communicating with others. ... I know that I live with them in a common world. Most importantly, I know that there is an ongoing correspondence between *my* meanings and *their* meanings in this world, that we share a common sense about its reality" (p. 23). Berger and Luckman are saying that an individual's everyday life is constructed by the individual and by the others in that individual's life—*together*. The strength of the individual's own unique identity is balanced by the equally powerful elements of a common world, a world shared with others.

The two dimensions of one's being, the unique and the shared, demand adjustment and readjustment throughout life. As Berger and Luckman (1966) stated, "The relationship between the individual and the objective social world is like an ongoing balancing act" (p. 134); because of this ongoing relationship, a person can only be wholly present and understood "*along with*" his or her social world (p. 132). This is another declaration, similar to Buber's (1958) philosophy that human beings dwell in relation. We are *who* we are because of forces that mold us from within and from without. We *are* only insofar as our form and our being are in connection with the world in which we live. In relation, we are wholly human beings.

## RELATION AND THE PROFESSIONAL

> I worked individually with a kid who was an extremely depressed adolescent and took him on as a special assistant ... to help establish some trust and bolster his esteem. I probably was not being objective enough. I don't know what it was about how really sick this kid was. Though I was not responsible for what happened, I felt badly, I think, because I couldn't remain objective about this case. The child killed himself, not while I was there, but he hung himself.

This quote is from an interview with an occupational therapist who was asked to think back over her practice and describe her most dissatisfying experience (Hasselkus & Dickie, 1994, raw data). The story is about an adolescent with whom she worked in therapy. As she continued to tell the story, the therapist described the different occupations that she enabled the teenager to take part in and the amount of time she spent with him:

> He worked with me in my group room as an assistant. We spent a lot of time [together], he helped me clean molds, and he helped me do things.

Hasselkus, B. R.
*The Meaning of Everyday Occupation, Second Edition* (pp. 103-122).
© 2011 SLACK Incorporated

We spent a lot of time just kind of talking. And he helped me assist another occupational therapist and physical therapy staff put on a play, and he was the stage manager and there was a lot of responsibility that he had.

The therapist ended the story by saying, "I felt good about what I did with him, but in the long run I felt very badly about the case and I have struggled with why for many years. ... Somehow the caretaker in me felt like I was going to be good enough to make it better and I've never worked through that particular part."

Near the beginning of the narrative, the therapist twice revealed what she thought was one of the things she did wrong—"I probably wasn't being objective enough" and "I felt badly because I couldn't remain objective." Her words conveyed the sense that she thought that her inability to "remain objective" had somehow contributed to the tragic ending of the story, that not being objective enough was part of the reason why she had not been "good enough to make it better."

This occupational therapist gave voice to the tension that exists within a clinician between maintaining a level of distance from the recipients of our therapy services and yet at the same time striving for a meaningful level of connection. The same kind of tension can exist between a therapist-researcher and the participants in his or her study. Loree Primeau, reflecting on her ethnographic research on work and play in families, wrote of her "dilemma" as a researcher—that is, "how to simultaneously strive for connection and rapport with my participants and yet minimize my intrusiveness and the inevitable effects of my presence on their daily life experiences" (2003, p. 13).

Cohn and Lyons (2003) expanded on the nature of tensions in the researcher–participant relationship, focusing on the ever-present struggle to find the right balance of power and the right presentation of self in the context of qualitative research. As an interviewer in a research project with people who had Parkinson's disease, Lyons wrote in her journal, "When the interview was over, they both [husband and wife] started asking me questions about myself—was I married, did I have children, was I involved in religious activity? I left feeling somewhat like an adopted granddaughter. ..." When Lyons called these participants later to schedule a second interview, "she [the wife] told me to bring my bathing suit so we could relax and visit in their pool after the interview ... What am I going to do? I think it would be odd and awkward if I took them up on the offer but I don't want to hurt their feelings by refusing ... I don't want them to think I am only interested in them as 'data-producing' research participants!" (p. 44). Lyon's quandary is an excellent example of the researcher's tension between maintaining a certain distance and objectivity while also developing meaningful connections (participants as "data" and/or feeling like an adopted granddaughter).

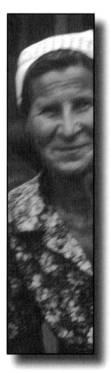

## Objectivism as Highly Valued

At least in Western society, we live in a world in which objectivism is highly valued (Palmer, 1987). *Objectivism* is defined as holding the world at a distance, keeping it at arm's length and apart from one's self so as to prevent contamination or bias from encroaching on the situations in which we are involved. In the eyes of the objectivist, the world is "out there" and it reflects "truth." As objectivists, we seek to know and analyze this truth. As Palmer said, "Once you have made something into an object … you can then chop that object up into pieces to see what makes it tick" (p. 22). You can analyze it, figure out what makes it work, and understand its various components. Ultimately, objectivism is experimental, that is, after we have dissected the world, we are then free to move the pieces around and reshape the world in other ways.

The therapist who related the dissatisfying narrative above felt that it was a failing on her part not to have been able to remain objective in her interactions with the troubled adolescent boy. Had she been able to remain objective, she seems to feel that she would have done a better job of understanding how sick he really was and then subsequently figuring out how to help him (i.e., how to "move the pieces around and reshape the world").

Palmer (1987) stated that people's capacities for relatedness with each other and with their worlds are constrained by the pervasive objectivist view. Because much of our society is imbued with and dominated by the values of objectivism, the distancing between knower and known tends to become also the distancing between the living person and his or her world. This constraint comprises another lifelong balancing act for human beings.

## A Shift Toward Relation?

Tension between a world of objectivity and a world of relation is the theme in a whole body of literature that emerged in the 1970s and 1980s (Capra, 1983; Ferguson, 1980; Kuhn, 1972; Naisbitt, 1982). According to Capra, the highly developed objectivist views of science, long held by Western society, have undergone a major shift—a turning point—in the latter part of the 20th century; relativity theory and quantum theory have shattered the previous view of the world as a huge machine. Quantum theory deals only with interconnections and relationships, not with objects or things. Human beings are a part of these relationships and the basic structures of the world are determined, ultimately, by the way we look at the world. Capra stated, "To put it bluntly, scientists do not deal with truth; they deal with limited and approximate descriptions of reality" (p. 48). Ferguson (1980) described the shift in thinking that is represented by this turning point as a "new knowing … a sense of awakening after being asleep" (p. 32). It is no small feat to make this shift; as one of my faculty colleagues said, "It's harder to expand one's paradigm than it is to shrink one's waistline!"

In the meantime, however, while the power of objectivism may be moderating, and intellectual and philosophical views of the world may be shifting toward relationship, other socially dynamic forces continue to contribute to people's tendencies to distance themselves from each other. According to Putnam (2000), who has written the book with the intriguing title *Bowling Alone,* social engagement, meaning activity that involves direct human contact, has been steadily declining over the second half of the past century. This decline includes all types of cultural or recreational activities such as churchgoing, card-playing, philanthropic men's and women's groups, or even just eating dinner together as a family. Activities that have increased are those that involve little or no human interaction such as watching television, going to movies, working at the computer, playing video games. Putnam has, thus, articulated another threat to "relation." One might predict that people's capacity for relatedness will wither on the vine if not exercised regularly within contexts of social engagement. The decline of activities with direct human contact and the rise of activities that involve no human contact are forces that impose another kind of constraint on human beings relatedness to each other. In Putnam's view, these occupational shifts are further sources of tension and constraint within relation in our lives. (Not all agree with Putnam's interpretation of current trends in social engagement in the United States; see Myers [2000] for a different view.)

The intent of providing this somewhat esoteric background information in this chapter on connectedness is to sharpen our awareness of the implicit assumptions and values that are part of Western culture. Without some understanding of the history of ideas, those ideas are sometimes presumed to be givens, all-time truths, instead of what they really are (i.e., part of our evolutionary thinking and knowledge about the world and our way of being in the world).

Centuries of objectivism have long convinced us that the only way to come to know something is through the scientific method—a method that only works if you objectify what you are addressing. This point is the source of anguish to the therapist who worked with the adolescent boy. Alternatively, in a relational view, the world is a reflection of our minds and the universe is a network of dynamic relationships. We *dwell* in our relation with others. We embrace subjectivity, not objectivity, as our way to come to know our worlds. Yet strong occupational forces seem to be pulling us toward activities that do not include human contact, that do not foster human relationships, but that are, rather, solitary activities that may require interaction only with technology.

# RELATION AND WELL-BEING

Connectedness and relatedness are generally thought of as positive states of being in ordinary everyday living. We refer to their opposites as *isolation, withdrawal,* or *being cut off, out of touch, distanced*; these are terms that have negative connotations in the context of daily life. To be connected is desirable; connectedness with one's self, one's surrounding world, and with a larger meaning or purpose in life is to be spiritually healthy (Bellingham, Cohen, Jones, & Spaniol, 1989). In our own literature, the occupational dimension of *belonging*—proposed as a basic human need—is a dimension of connection and relatedness (Hammell, 2004; Wilcock, 2006).

## Social Support Theory

A large literature exists on what is called *social networks* and *social support theory*; that is, the theory of the effects of the quantity, quality, and function of people's social relationships on their mortality and morbidity (see, for example, Hupcey, 1998; Rosengren, Orth-Gomer, Wedel, & Wilhelmsen, 1993; Ståhl et al., 2001). Much of this research supports social relationships as mediators of stress, sickness, and death. Social relationships are a strong component of social connectedness and a symbol of living "in relation" in our society.

Cobb (1976), one of the early proponents of social support theory, stated, "It appears that social support can protect people in crisis from a wide variety of pathological states: from low birth weight to death, from arthritis through tuberculosis to depression, alcoholism, and the social breakdown syndrome. Furthermore, social support may reduce the amount of medication required, accelerate recovery, and facilitate compliance with prescribed medical regimens" (p. 300). Both the *structure* of the social network (frequency of social contacts, duration of contacts, number of people in the social network) and the *quality and function* of social support (the strength of the relationship, the reciprocity, the helping behaviors themselves) have been studied as they relate to health (Hupcey, 1998).

Despite Cobb's (1976) strong claim regarding the moderating effects of social support on stress, health, and health care behaviors, empirical evidence to support these claims has not been unequivocal (see Avlund, Damsgaard, & Holstein [1998] for a good review of social support research since the 1970s). Early research seemed to show strong relationships between mortality and the structure of the networks (e.g., Berkman, 1984; Blazer, 1982). This is the body of research that led to the well-accepted (and well-supported) axiom that living alone is a high risk factor for morbidity and mortality. More and more, recent research seems to recognize the complexity and nuances of the concept of social support; important influences such as gender (Avlund et al.), culture (Sugisawa, Liang, & Liu, 1994), and type of social participation (Glass, de Leon, Marottoli, & Berkman, 1999) are being incorporated into research designs. The broad sweeping claims of Cobb, as quoted above, have been tempered by often conflicting findings in this body of research.

The conflicting findings of the social support research serve as reminders to us that we have only just begun to comprehend the meanings of being "in relation" in our lives. The relation itself is not embodied in the frequency of social contacts, in the length of time spent with others, in the number of people in one's intimate social circle; nor is

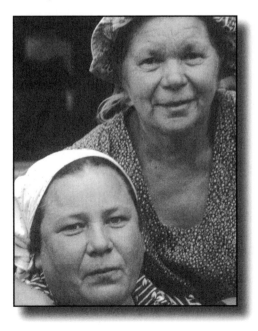

relation embodied in the actions taken or the emotional depth felt toward another person. These may be manifestations of relation, but they are not relation itself.

## *Too Much Connectedness?*

While writing this chapter for the first edition of this book, I was startled one morning by a small headline in the newspaper. A column written by *New York Times* writer Thomas L. Friedman (1999) was headlined, "Yes, You Can Be Too Connected." Reading the article under the headline further strengthened my increasing awareness that relation or connectedness is not a simple, unidimensional phenomenon; rather it is an aspect of life that harbors destructive as well as supportive potentialities.

In the newspaper article, Friedman (1999) wrote that overconnectedness will be the "social disease of the next millennium." He expounded on people's increasingly common expectations that we can always be within reach of each other, no matter where we are. Obviously, this ready accessibility has increased exponentially since 1999 with high-tech cell phones, e-mail, text messaging, Twitter, Facebook, MySpace, answering machines, voice mail, and more. Friedman called this way of life a "virus of overconnectedness" which, he said, is "spreading daily, and it has no known cure." Now, when people are trying to reach us, we are never "out"—we just need to be reached in another way. Friedman continued, "Out is over. Now, you're always in. And when you're always in, you're always on. And when you're always on, you're just like a computer server. You can never stop and relax."

I was somewhat taken aback by this small article. Up to this point, I had been headed toward a chapter that covered the capacities of occupation to enhance and facilitate connectedness. My research has been on caregiving for people with dementia, and the bridges that occupation helps build between people with dementia and their worlds can be beautiful to behold (Hasselkus, 1998). Also, up to this point I had been thinking of technology from Putnam's (2000) point of view, as a source of *dis*connection from involvement in human contact. But this newspaper article expanded my thinking. Of *course* one can be too connected. And of course the concept of human connection is complex and has many dimensions; it is a mistake to reduce the many possible forms of human interaction to only this or only that. And, as with so much of what we experience in life, the *balance* of it all is what makes the difference.

## A Balance of Solitude and Relation

There is a Buddhist saying that it is always a mistake to think your soul can go it alone. Yet it is also inconceivable to think of being in the presence of others all the time. May Sarton was a poet and novelist who published a series of five personal journals in the later years of her life. Sarton struggled throughout life to achieve a balance between solitude and social connection. Her journals are not chronicles of events and happenings in her life, but rather they are compelling presentations of the inner experiences of her day-to-day life. In her first journal, *Journal of a Solitude*, written at the age of 59, Sarton wrote of the importance of separateness in her life. After a spate of days full of visitors and busy-ness with other people, Sarton wrote, "I am here alone for the first time in weeks to take up my 'real life' again at last" (1973, p. 11). Then she expanded on this experience of aloneness, remarking on a closeness she felt to other parts of her world when she was in solitude: "When I am alone the flowers are really seen; I can pay attention to them. They are felt presences" (p. 11).

In her 1980 journal, *Recovering: A Journal*, Sarton acknowledged the power of both separateness and attachment in her reflections during a year of recovery after a stroke: "The two greatest yearnings of humans may be the yearnings for inclusion and the yearnings for distinctness" (p. 142). She expressed a need for both, as both contributed importantly to her sense of self and her ability to *be* herself in her daily life.

The balance in social relationship that we strive for is not simply a matter of finding parity between being alone and being with others; to be alone does not necessarily constitute being out of relation or disconnected, and to be with others does not necessarily

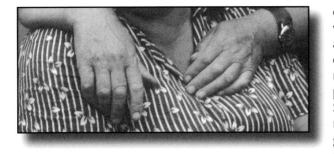

constitute connectedness. It is what takes place within that aloneness or that being with others that signifies whether relation or lack of relation is present. In aloneness, May Sarton felt much more connected to the flowers in her garden than she did when she had other people present. When she was alone, the flowers were "really seen" and they were "felt presences." In other words, Sarton felt *closer* to some parts of her immediate world when she was alone. Her experience of aloneness was not one of withdrawal or isolation. In her aloneness, May Sarton was experiencing a different form of connectedness.

## OCCUPATIONAL FORMS OF RELATION

Occupation offers us a powerful way to develop and maintain a balance of relation in day-to-day living. Whiteford (2007) explored how occupation connects us with others in our world and provides us with a sense of continuity in our lives. Occupation can be a deterrent or an enhancer of connectedness in the world. With each of these capacities, occupation can contribute positively or negatively to a person's well-being.

I remember a spirited discussion in a graduate student seminar generated by reading the published version of Anne Wilcock's keynote speech given in Montreal at the 1998 World Federation of Occupational Therapists Congress (Wilcock, 1998). Wilcock made the statement that "what people *do* creates and shapes the societies in which we live *for good or bad*" (p. 250, emphasis added). Further, she pointed out that we have "scant research to date about how *doing* may be injurious to health and well-being" (p. 250). In other words, the emphasis in occupational therapy research and practice has been almost solely on how occupation is related to the "good"—to health and well-being. Wilcock's notion of defining occupation potentially as doing good *or* bad was at first unpalatable to several graduate students in the seminar; they wanted occupation to be, by definition, only that which leads to healthful outcomes. In reality, surely occupation can be either for "good or bad"; one has only to think of high-risk behaviors such as gang memberships or drug use or anorexia to recognize harmful occupations. As it relates to relation and connectedness, occupation can be a constraint or a facilitator, and both of those attributes can either enhance or diminish well-being.

The duality of occupation as harbinger of "good" or "bad" is well illustrated in an experience shared with me by a daycare staff person for my research on the meaning of activity for people with dementia. The story she told focuses on a participant at the daycare center and the occupation "eating"—a self-care activity prominent in many areas of occupational therapy practice:

> This particular client would become very agitated being with the group, especially at mealtime. And he was not eating well. What we suggested doing was to bring him back into the office area where it's somewhat more

quiet. … And when he would be in a quiet, more controlled situation, he just did very well. … He would actually sit down with his meal and bless himself and his food. … He ate much better and he was even concerned if he would spill something, and just seemed to be *much more in touch with reality* (Hasselkus, 1998, p. 428, emphasis added).

For this daycare center client, to be in the room with many other people during mealtime was to be very *dis*connected—from the other people, from the task of eating the meal, from the occupation of mealtime. Alternatively, to be by himself, away from other people, was to be much more connected with the task itself ("he was even concerned if he would spill something") and with the occupation of mealtime ("he ate much better and he would actually sit down with his meal and bless himself and his food"). The former situation surely represents occupation as being potentially injurious, the latter represents occupation as enhancing health and well-being. Obviously, the daycare staff person used her skills to shift the occupational form in such a way as to bring about better connections between the participant and his world. Also, as this story clearly illustrates (as did May Sarton's journal entry), being connected does not necessarily mean being in the company of other people; for this daycare client, being in a room by himself meant being "much more in touch with reality."

## Occupation and Connection to One's World

Of course, occupation can also be the catalyst that enhances connection between people. The doing of occupation can forge connections among people and forging connections with other people can lead to the doing of occupation. Both represent the heart of occupational therapy theory—using occupation to bring about wellness, to help people be connected to their worlds.

Such was the case in a staff experience with a person with dementia at the same daycare center. The staff member described what she perceived as rather remarkable participation by one client brought about by a group activity:

> We were doing a read-aloud reminisce-type activity, and one of our dementia clients, who usually doesn't actively participate in a read-aloud, kind of just took it upon herself to read right out of one of the magazines and turned it into her own little discussion … and maybe because she grew up on a farm, I thought, you know, that it caught her eye. The article was "Why are Barns Painted Red?" And then we sat around and we talked about it, and then she went on to read why barns are painted red. … Usually it will just be the staff doing the read-aloud, or you know, usually they won't read right out of a magazine out loud like that with the whole group, you know? And to turn it into a discussion, you know, on her own, she just kind of took it upon herself.

In my research (Hasselkus, 1998), *relative well-being* is a term I borrowed from Kitwood and Bredin (1992) to describe the results of this kind of engagement in occupation by a person with dementia. For the woman in the above story, relative well-being meant attending to an activity for a period of time, spontaneously engaging in the activity, and relating directly to other people as she carried out the activity. Being in the group led to occupational participation and the occupation of "doing the read-aloud" forged connections between the woman with dementia and other people in the group. Whiteford would call this connection "community engagement" (2007, p. 77), in this case a *localized* community engagement.

Perhaps the most obvious real-life experiences of connection through occupation are those of children and their play experiences. In Miller and Kuhaneck's study (2008) of children's perceptions of play experiences, "fun" emerged as the core category that explained choice of play activities. One key subtheme within fun was relational; "The relational aspects of play involved whom to play with and who decided what to play. … All the children preferred to play with others rather than alone and felt that play was more fun with their peers" (p. 411). Further, related to play preferences and choices, fun was more important than other specific play characteristics such as who got to make the play choice or whether the person played with was child or adult. Since play is used in therapy as both a developmental measure and an intervention, the authors felt that the relational dimension of fun tapped into the children's intrinsic motivations and could be a useful understanding for therapists as they make choices for therapeutic activities.

## The Therapeutic Relationship as Connectedness

The therapeutic relationship is one form of connection between people that we, as a profession, highly value, although it is also an aspect of practice for which we feel inadequately prepared (Taylor, Lee, Kielhofner, & Ketkar, 2009). As therapists, we are hopeful that an occupational "good" will be the outcome of that relationship. As medical sociologist Schön (1983) has stated, professional–client relationships are primary sources of meaning for professionals in practice.

In my graduate student's phenomenological research on the meaning of therapist–patient relationships (Rosa & Hasselkus, 1996), "connecting with patients" emerged from the data as the central core theme of the stories shared by the therapists in the study (p. 247). The major subthemes of "helping" and "working together" reflected meanings that contributed to the therapists' sense of connection and to their experiences of satisfaction in practice. One therapist in the study told the story of a 14-year-old girl who was a burn patient:

> She was pretty hard [to work with] at first; as you probably know—burns—it is just so painful. We had a hard time getting her to do things or letting us do things with her. … It's probably been more since she's been an outpatient that we've just really built a relationship, I guess more established a good rapport, and I guess I'm seen more as a friend. She looks forward to coming to therapy but yet we still get done what we need to get done and we've ended up making quite a bit of improvement to where she's able to use her hand now. … I'm going to be moving in three months and she was almost in tears when I told her. She's like, "Well, can I come and visit you?" She's just really gotten invested as far as with the relationship and doing things in therapy. … I guess that's probably been the most gratifying experience.

The clear focus on the therapist-patient relationship as the "key" to bringing about improvement in the patient's ability to use her hand and the strong sense of connection between the therapist and patient can be seen in this narrative.

In the absence of helping and working together, the therapists who participated in the above study experienced dissatisfaction. A therapist in a psychiatric setting described her group work with patients as follows:

> Groups of patients were escorted to my craft clinic from various psychiatric wards for one-hour periods. One group from the geriatric infirm ward was usually 25 to 40 patients. Because of the size of this group, individual attention was brief or impossible. … There was little opportunity to develop therapeutic relationships. … In only a few cases did I feel that I was able to make any contribution to the well-being of these men or help in the relief of symptoms or the healing process. … I was very frustrated by working with this group and felt I was not making any impact and not really using my occupational therapy training or even interpersonal skills.

In this situation, although a form of occupation took place within the group activity program, the absence of therapeutic relationships in conjunction with that occupation left the therapist feeling very frustrated and unable "to make any contribution to the well-being of these men." This therapist's statements speak strongly to the key role that connecting and relation plays in the therapeutic process; without it, little therapeutic value is felt to be present in the situation.

Working together with someone, in a cooperative relationship, has been referred to as a form of *co-occupation* (Zemke & Clark, 1996); that is, occupation that requires the involvement of more than one person. In co-occupation, both people are seen as active participants in the activity; neither person is relegated to the position of being simply a passive observer or recipient of the occupation of the other. The sense of connection between client and therapist in a therapeutic relationship can be considered a form of co-occupation.

But therapeutic relationships are not so unidimensional as to be characterized by a single term such as co-occupation. In their discussion of clinical reasoning, Mattingly and Fleming (1994b) proposed the term *interactive reasoning* to describe the collaborative thinking that occurs when therapist and client work together (p. 178). Presumably interactive reasoning is a process that helps to bring about engagement in co-occupation. Another related concept—*client-centered care*—was introduced in Canada in 1983 (Department of National Health & Welfare); scholarly works using this term (also, *enabling occupation*) emerged in subsequent years (Law, 1998a; Law, Baptiste, & Mills, 1995; Townsend, Langille, & Ripley, 2003). Key principles of client-centered care include client autonomy, partnership, shared responsibility, and respect for diversity. The ideal of client-centered practice is one in which therapy is directed by clients' own decisions and priorities rather than by the therapist-generated goals and treatment. The realization of this ideal likely requires a major shift in

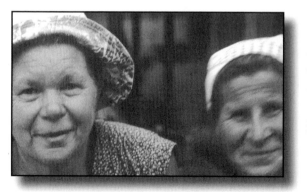

therapeutic practice away from the therapist-directed process that has been tradition-ally experienced.

The term *family-centered care* has also come to the fore within the profession (Law, 1998b). Proponents of this term like the way it expands our thinking beyond one-to-one therapy with an individual patient or client to consideration of a client only within his or her larger social context. Occupational therapy literature with a family focus is reflected in research such as that on children and parents (Bedell, Cohn, & Dumas, 2005; Primeau, 2000; Stewart & Meyer, 2004), on caregivers for people with mul-tiple sclerosis (McKeown, Porter-Armstrong, & Baxter, 2004), and research on elderly clients, their family caregivers and grandparenting occupations (Gitlin, Corcoran, & Leinmiller-Eckhardt, 1995; Hasselkus & Murray, 2007; Ludwig, Hattjar, Russell, & Winston, 2007).

The literature on therapeutic relationships in occupational therapy also uses the metaphor of shared stories to convey the nature of therapist-client relationships (Crepeau, 1991; Hasselkus & Dickie, 1994; Helfrich, Kielhofner, & Mattingly, 1994; Kautzman, 1993; Mattingly & Fleming, 1994a; Peloquin, 1993; Rosa & Hasselkus, 1996, 2005; Taylor et al., 2009). In my work with Virginia Dickie (Hasselkus & Dickie, 1994), relationships with clients, team members, and family caregivers emerged as a primary theme of meaning in the stories about satisfying and dissatisfying practice gathered from occupational therapists nationwide. In the analysis of all the interview data, we labeled the theme of relationships as Community. We stated the following: "We imagine that community in therapy evolves as people's stories become superim-posed on each other, in effect as a new story is created. ... In the stories of satisfying Community, the therapist describes with enthusiasm how well people worked together. The actors in the story have created shared beliefs and expectations, mutual views of the present, and hopes for the future" (p. 149). In contrast, the stories of dissatisfying Community were those in which the beliefs and expectations of the therapist, patient, and others were discordant, with each person vying for command of the new story.

Grady, in her 1994 Eleanor Clark Slagle Lecture (Grady, 1995), challenged occupational therapists to "promote more interactive models of practice" (p. 300) in order to build a sense of inclusiveness and community in therapy; she defined inclusiveness and community as contexts that honor both individual potential and oneness with others; that is, that which is unique and that which is shared. Thus, community means maintaining our individuality while sustaining our connectedness with the world around us. Community represents the *balance* of connectedness discussed in this chapter, the balance that is needed to sustain health and well-being during our work together on this earth.

# OCCUPATIONAL THERAPY
# AND CONNECTEDNESS

In many ways, Western medical care is characterized by a deep and broad objectiv-ism. The "diagnose, treat, and cure" approach to medical care that we are so familiar with today is deeply entrenched in the values of objectivism—the reliance on norms as guidelines for interpreting behaviors, symptoms, treatments, and responses; the division of the person into parts—first, mind and body, and, then, all the components of each of these (the id, ego, and superego; body systems, body organs, cellular and molecular structures); and finally, the health care professional's attempts to "rearrange" the mind or body of the "other" so as to bring about a return to health. These are the values and skills that the occupational therapist felt were missing in her therapy with the adolescent boy who was depressed. Her idealism regarding an objectivist approach to therapy is apparent in her rapprochement of herself for not being "objective enough" and for not being able "to make it better."

Back in 1976, arch-critic Ivan Illich wrote in his *The Limits to Medicine: Medical Nemesis—The Expropriation of Health* that health care had become "an engineering endeavor that has translated human survival from the performance of organisms into the result of technical manipulation" (p. 7). Waitzkin (1991), political analyst of medicine in the United States, has observed that technical statements in health care discourse convert health problems into objects; "Symptoms, signs, and treatments take on an aura of scientific fact, rather than of subjective manifestations of a troubled social reality" (p. 16). Now, as we experience the new millennium, the manipulative potential of technology in health care has surely increased many times over.

## The Two-Body Practice in Occupational Therapy

Objectivism in our occupational therapy practice is evident in the standardized assessments that we urge therapists to use, in our practice focus on body systems and body parts, and in our efforts to change our clients with the application of various treatments. Objectivism has served our profession well in many ways as we have developed our discipline and credibility in the health care world. But this kind of thinking is a problem if we are trying to promote a balance of detachment and relatedness. Objectivism is the antithesis of relatedness. Objectivism is distancing, breaking the whole down into separate parts, manipulating the parts into new configurations. Objectivism reflects an "us and them" kind of world; it is a world with me over here and you over there; it is I observing you and you being observed by me (Kitwood & Bredin, 1992).

Much of Peloquin's work has focused on alerting the profession to the tendency of all health professionals to depersonalize patients, and to fail to recognize or acknowledge the power of empathy and the strength of affective meanings in our work (Peloquin, 1993, 1995, 2002). For more than a decade, Peloquin's writings have given "voice" to relatedness and affective aspects of the therapeutic process as she has strived to capture the attention of the profession and gain recognition for what she believes to be the most important aspect of occupational therapy.

Occupational therapists are caught up in a balancing act as they strive to function both within the dominant health care paradigm of the human body as a machine and within the newly emerging paradigm of the human body as lived experience. Cheryl Mattingly (1994) called occupational therapy a "two-body practice" (p. 37). One practice addresses the body as machine, relying heavily on a biomedical framework for its expression and structure; this is the practice that tends to address the body and its components as separable entities, that treats disability and its symptoms as though they can be separated out from the person and the person's life context. The second practice addresses the body as a lived body, relying on phenomenological views of the body as part of a person's experiences in the world; that is, a view of the body in relation to the world. In the phenomenological view, disabilities are viewed as lived experiences; the body, itself, is part of the world that the person brings with him or her. Mattingly stated, "Sometimes therapists are able to synthesize these two ways of understanding disability in an effective way, and sometimes they have trouble integrating the two perspectives" (p. 39). Occupational therapists' capacities for relatedness are the result of the ongoing negotiation of the tension between these cultural forces.

To synthesize the objective and experiential views of illness and disability into one integrated perspective is no easy feat. In our study of satisfying and dissatisfying experiences of doing occupational therapy (Hasselkus & Dickie, 1994), one occupational therapist told the story of her work with a group of female adolescents who had "a lot of behavioral problems." The setting was a state psychiatric facility, and part of what the staff worked toward was helping the girls to learn appropriate ways to communicate their needs, to understand sexuality issues, and to learn to work cooperatively at an age-appropriate level in a group. These goals seem to be drawing from the biomedical view of health, breaking life down into individual skills and teaching those skills for living—representing one "body" of the two-body practice. Yet, the other body—that which represents the girls' lived experiences in the world—was also part of this practice. The therapist described the group project as follows:

> They were feeling the lack of ability to work and earn money for themselves to buy Christmas presents for their families. … So they set some goals for themselves to do some projects—baking and raising plants and craft projects—and have a sale. … We had this group of about six girls who worked pretty solidly together and they planned meals every week and learned to do some cooking and we went shopping and learned to do some grocery shopping and menu planning and all those kind of nutritional and exploratory things that you'd like to see adolescents begin. … and so they ended up learning to make stuff for the bake sale. And we raised plants from seeds and from cuttings and had our own horticulture area that we spent some time in weekly. So they raised plants and they did pottery and ceramics and macramé. … and we set up in the lobby with permission from the administration to put on a sale that went for two days and the girls actually acted as the sales clerks and in a two-day sale, they raised over $300.
>
> The long shot of it was that at the end of it they felt very good about themselves. They had control, they had the ability to make decisions, they learned to work through some conflicts, they learned how to communicate better with their parents. … There was a real group cohesiveness in the sense of companionship that I think would have been difficult to achieve with that group had they been at home, and certainly would have been difficult to do with them in a hospital setting. … It was something that really felt good to me.

To me, this is a story of a therapist who was able to synthesize the two-body practice—she was able to understand the objectivist view of disability so that she could set measurable goals and work with the girls on specific skills, but she was also able to understand the phenomenological view of practice; that is, to create for these girls lived experiences that helped them build relationships and engage in everyday meaningful occupations.

## Ideology of Independence

"In the beginning of life, when we are infants, we need others to survive, right? And at the end of life, when you get like me, you need others to survive, right?" His voice dropped to a whisper. "But here's the secret: in between we need others as well" (Albom, 1997, p. 157; words spoken by Morrie near the end of his life).

Another source of tension between occupational therapists and the phenomenon of relation is derived from the rehabilitation ideology of independence. An ideology is a "set of ideas and doctrines that form the distinctive perspective of a social group" (Waitzkin, 1991, p. 12). One prominent ideology in Western society is the strong valuing placed on individual initiative and accomplishments, on self-sufficiency, and on rugged individualism (Myers, 2000). In our social culture, we admire the person who works hard, who doesn't give up, who overcomes obstacles by persistence and "stick-to-it-iveness." In the context of rehabilitation, these ideologies are reproduced as goals for individual independence in the everyday activities of life and as expectations for patient behaviors that reflect individual initiative, personal responsibility, and perseverance (Becker & Kaufman, 1995). In the context of society, Myers asserted that these ideologies have eroded our civility as a people, and that we need to shift (and we actually are shifting) our social framework away from an emphasis on personal rights toward a more community orientation. We are recognizing that "in between we need others as well."

It can be readily seen that a tension exists between Western rehabilitation goals for independence and the concept of living in relation. Relation is being *with* others, feeling connected with one's world; independence is more acting with*out* others, functioning separately from others, using personal initiative. In a contrasting Eastern philosophy, Iwama (2005) has presented the Japanese Kawa (river) model of "how one constructs the world and situates the self in relation to it" (p. 217). In the Kawa model, "Life is a complex, profound journey that flows through time and space like a river" (p. 218). The self is not construed as a central privileged entity separate from the whole of the world, but is, rather, "merely one integrated part of a greater universe," no greater and no less than all other aspects of our social and material environments (Iwama). Harmony or balance in life is conceptualized as life flow; occupational therapy's purpose in this Eastern model is to help patients and clients "enhance or balance this flow" (p. 217).

In Western ideology, the tension between relation and independence is dramatically illustrated in a study of dependent behaviors among residents in a nursing home (Baltes, 1988). Baltes studied the naturally occurring social conditions that surround dependent and independent behaviors by nursing home residents during their daily activities. In her review of research on patterns of behavior, Baltes found that, among elderly people in institutions, "dependent self-care behaviors are followed by a high amount of social action, while independent self-care behaviors are not" (p. 307). In other words, the dominant response by institutional staff to a resident's independent behaviors is *no* response; independent behaviors do not generate social interactions. Dependent self-care behaviors, on the other hand, have the *highest* probability of being followed by attention and social interaction from others in the institutional environment.

Baltes' (1998) research clearly reveals the tension between independence and social relation. If independent self-care behavior is followed by little or no response from the people in one's environment, and if one is residing in an environment where opportunities for meaningful social interaction are especially rare, then what is the motivation for being independent when it is simply a guarantee for further isolation from the others in the environment? The pattern of behavioral sequences reported by Baltes provides evidence for powerful pathways of influence between the environment and behavior.

In some health care situations, dependent *and* independent behaviors generate social interaction. For example, in my research on family caregivers for elderly family members in the community, one caregiver described her approach to caring for her husband who had experienced a stroke as follows: "The therapist said to never let him fall. So, when he gets up [out of the wheelchair], I get up. 'Cuz I wouldn't want him to fall and break a hip or something—then I couldn't take care of him and I don't want him to have to go to a nursing home" (Hasselkus, 1991). In this situation, attempts by the husband to get up and move about independently were viewed as full of risk; the caregiver's strategy was to keep a vigilant watch on her husband's actions and to quickly move to his side whenever he started to get up. This is an example of social interaction following *in*dependent behavior. The situation represents the potential ethical dilemma imposed by the moral need to both ensure a person's safety and at the same time respect his or her autonomy (Collopy, 1995).

These examples of patterns of social interaction make it clear that social connectedness and occupation are intimately related, with each inseparable from the other in many different ways. These influences may or may not be health promoting for the individuals involved in the social situation— it depends. In applying the Kawa (river) model to these examples, one could say that the life flow is out of balance in each situation, and harmony of the subject—within and inseparable from the context—is compromised. An occupational therapist in each situation would seek to establish a more balanced life flow.

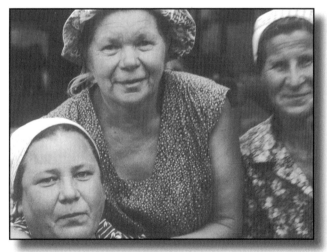

## *Relation and Well-Being in Institutional Settings*

It may seem paradoxical that, for people who live in institutionalized settings (e.g., nursing homes, group homes, assisted living facilities), where other people are in close proximity all of the time, having private rather than shared rooms may actually increase the amount of daily social interaction that takes place (Ward, 1984). Social withdrawal can be a response to situations that lack privacy. Having one's own room presumably offers a person a sense of choice and perhaps control that can offset the population density and potential over-connectedness of the group living situation. Having a room of one's own may enable a person to reconnect with family and the past through books, letters, pictures, music, moments of undistracted thought; receiving a visitor on one's "own" territory may enhance the possibility of meaningful exchange and connection during the interaction.

Mitchell and Kemp (2000) studied quality of life in assisted living homes and found that a cohesive social environment—measured by how supportive staff members were toward residents and how supportive residents were toward each other—was the strongest predictor of quality of life for the residents. At first glance, this finding may seem at odds with the point just made about providing opportunities for solitude in group-living facilities. Yet, along with the importance of cohesion were other predictors, such as family contact and an environment low in conflict. In their conclusions, the authors stated, "… a more homelike and warm environment with a less conflictual setting is the key to contented residents and QOL [Quality of Life] along with both family and social involvement" (p. P125). To me, a "more homelike" environment includes—*minimally*—having a room to call one's own, having a say in decisions about how one wants to spend the day, and having flexibility and freedom from too many rules and regulations in as many aspects of one's life as possible.

In an alternative institutional setting, Finlayson and her colleagues (Finlayson, Baker, Rodman, & Herzberg, 2002) conducted a needs assessment at a homeless shelter, focusing initially on the needs of the individual residents. By the end of the study, they had broadened their attention to include the staff and the organization of the shelter; the "discordance between staff and resident priorities and the negative influences of the organizational structure" (p. 319) led to expanded thinking and involvement in the agency. For example, whereas the residents' goals were "finding some meaning and direction in their lives," the staff focused on "finding jobs for the residents and moving them out of the shelter" (p. 318); staff were "incredulous" to learn that some of the residents did not see themselves as homeless because they considered the shelter their home. Organizational policy meant that a fairly large number of residents (two dozen at the time of the study) stayed in the shelter during the day because of mental illness or other disabilities; "no programming was provided for these persons, and few resources or materials were available to help them fill their days" (p. 317). The need for connection and relationship-building between staff and residents was revealed over and over in the study; mediation between staff and residents and help in sharing information with each other (connection!) became new priorities. For the research team, the study took on the characteristics of a "situational diagnosis" (as introduced in chapter 2), informed by the power structures within the organization, and the need for negotiation and definition of boundaries (Watson, 2004).

In an institutional setting, the balance between meaningful connections with others and one's immediate surroundings as well as meaningful opportunities to be alone may need to be thoughtfully facilitated through opportunities for solitude as well as group projects. Otherwise, a person may feel that he or she is merely part of a "lonely crowd."

In the poem "A Hermit Thrush" by Amy Clampitt (1987), two lines read as follows: "... and all attachment may prove at best, perhaps, a broken, a much-mended thing" (p. 101). Connection is not a thing to be taken for granted. We must keep creating and mending our attachments to our world, for connection is not a static, stable state of being; instead, connection is a dynamic, responsive, fluctuating and sometimes fragile phenomenon. Being aware of the historically strong ideologies of our Western society and health care systems increases our awareness of the social forces that work against connection and relation. The Japanese Kawa (river) model provides an Eastern philosophy of the oneness of self with the world and the goal of reaching harmony in the life flow of our lives. At the same time, the late 20th and early 21st centuries have brought technological opportunities to our world that may put us at risk for too much electronic connectedness in our lives and too little connectedness through direct human contact. Occupation can serve as a catalyst to enhance meaningful connection with our worlds or to moderate and constrain connection; either enhancement or constraint can be supportive of a person's health and well-being, depending on the circumstances. It is the balance of connectedness and separation that we seek. Occupation is a therapeutic resource for achieving that balance.

# REFERENCES

Albom, M. (1997). *Tuesdays with Morrie: An old man, a young man, and life's greatest lesson.* New York, NY: Doubleday.

Avlund, K., Damsgaard, M. T., & Holstein, B. E. (1998). Social relationships and mortality: An eleven year follow-up study of 70-year-old men and women in Denmark. *Social Science & Medicine, 47,* 635-643.

Baltes, M. M. (1988). The etiology and maintenance of dependency in the elderly: Three phases of operant research. *Behavior Therapy, 19,* 301-319.

Becker, G., & Kaufman, S. (1995). Managing an uncertain illness trajectory in old age: Patients' and physicians' views of stroke. *Medical Anthropology Quarterly, 9,* 165-187.

Bedell, G. M., Cohn, E. S., & Dumas, H. M. (2005). Exploring parents' use of strategies to promote social participation of school-age children with acquired brain injuries. *American Journal of Occupational Therapy, 59,* 273-284.

Bellingham, R., Cohen, B., Jones, T., & Spaniol, L. (1989). Connectedness: Some skills for spiritual health. *American Journal of Health Promotion, 4,* 18-24.

Berger, P. L., & Luckman, T. (1966). *The social construction of reality.* New York, NY: Doubleday.

Berkman, L. F. (1984). Assessing the physical health effects of social networks and social support. *Annual Review of Public Health, 5,* 413-432.

Blazer, D. G. (1982). Social support and mortality in an elderly community population. *American Journal of Epidemiology, 115,* 684-694.

Buber, M. (1958). *I and thou* (R. G. Smith, Trans.). New York, NY: Macmillan.

Capra, F. (1983). *The turning point.* New York, NY: Bantam Books.

Clampitt, A. (1987). *Archaic figure.* New York, NY: Alfred A. Knopf.

Cobb, S. (1976). Social support as a moderator of life stress. *Psychosomatic Medicine, 38,* 300-314.

Cohn, E. S., & Lyons, K. D. (2003). The perils of power in interpretive research. *American Journal of Occupational Therapy, 57,* 40-48.

Collopy, B. J. (1995). Safety and independence: Rethinking some basic concepts in long-term care. In L. B. McCullough & N. L. Wilson (Eds.), *Long-term care decisions: Ethical and conceptual dimensions*. Baltimore, MD: Johns Hopkins University Press.

Crepeau, E. (1991). Achieving intersubjective understanding: Examples from an occupational therapy treatment session. *American Journal of Occupational Therapy, 45*, 1016-1025.

Department of National Health and Welfare (1983). *Guidelines for the client-centred practice of occupational therapy*. Ottawa, Ontario, Canada: Minister of Supply and Services Canada.

Ferguson, M. (1980). *The aquarian conspiracy: Personal and social transformation in the 1980s*. Los Angeles, CA: J. P. Tarcher.

Finlayson, M., Baker, M., Rodman, L., & Herzberg, G. (2002). The process and outcomes of a multimethod needs assessment at a homeless shelter. *American Journal of Occupational Therapy, 56*, 313-321.

Friedman, T. L. (1999, August). Yes, you can be too connected. *New York Times*.

Gitlin, L. N., Corcoran, M., & Leinmiller-Eckhardt, S. (1995). Understanding the family perspective: An ethnographic framework for providing occupational therapy in the home. *American Journal of Occupational Therapy, 49*, 802-809.

Glass, T. A., de Leon, C. M., Marottoli, R. A., & Berkman, L. F. (1999). Population-based study of social and productive activities as predictors of survival among elderly Americans. *British Medical Journal, 319*, 478-483.

Grady, A. P. (1995). Building inclusive community: A challenge for occupational therapy. *American Journal of Occupational Therapy, 49*, 300-310.

Hammell, K. W. (2004). Dimensions of meaning in the occupations of daily life. *Canadian Journal of Occupational Therapy, 71*, 296-305.

Hasselkus, B. R. (1991). Ethical dilemmas: The organization of family caregiving for the elderly. *Journal of Aging Studies, 5*, 99-110.

Hasselkus, B. R. (1998). Occupation and well-being in dementia: The experience of daycare staff. *American Journal of Occupational Therapy, 52*, 423-434.

Hasselkus, B. R., & Dickie, V. A. (1994). Doing occupational therapy: Dimensions of satisfaction and dissatisfaction. *American Journal of Occupational Therapy, 48*, 145-154.

Hasselkus, B. R., & Murray, B. J. (2007). Everyday occupation, well-being and identity: The experience of caregivers in families with dementia. *American Journal of Occupational Therapy, 61*, 9-20.

Helfrich, C., Kielhofner, G., & Mattingly, C. (1994). Volition as narrative: Understanding motivation in chronic illness. *American Journal of Occupational Therapy, 48*, 311-318.

Hupcey, J. E. (1998). Social support: Assessing conceptual coherence. *Qualitative Health Research, 8*, 304-318.

Illich, I. (1976). *Medical nemesis: The expropriation of health*. New York, NY: Pantheon Books.

Iwama, M. K. (2005). The Kawa (river) model: Nature, life flow, and the power of culturally relevant occupational therapy. In F. Kronenberg, S. S. Algado, & N. Pollard (Eds.), *Occupational therapy without borders: Learning from the spirit of survivors* (pp. 213-227). London, UK: Elsevier.

Kautzmann, L. N. (1993). Linking patient and family stories to caregivers' use of clinical reasoning. *American Journal of Occupational Therapy, 47*, 169-173.

Kitwood, T., & Bredin, K. (1992). Towards a theory of dementia care: Personhood and well-being. *Aging and Society, 12*, 269-287.

Kuhn, T. S. (1972). *The structure of scientific revolutions*. Chicago, IL: University of Chicago Press.

Law, M. (1998a). *Client-centered occupational therapy*. Thorofare, NJ: SLACK Incorporated.

Law, M. (Ed.). (1998b). *Family-centred assessment and intervention in pediatric rehabilitation*. Binghamton, NY: Haworth Press.

Law, M., Baptiste, S., & Mills, J. (1995). Client-centred practice: What does it mean and does it make a difference? *Canadian Journal of Occupational Therapy, 62*, 250-257.

Ludwig, F. M., Hattjar, B., Russell, R. L., & Winston, W. (2007). How caregiving for grandchildren affects grandmothers' meaningful occupations. *Journal of Occupational Science, 14,* 40-51.

Mattingly, C. (1994). Occupational therapy as a two-body practice. In C. Mattingly & M. Fleming (Eds.), *Clinical reasoning: Forms of inquiry in a therapeutic practice* (pp. 37-93). Philadelphia, PA: F. A. Davis.

Mattingly, C., & Fleming, M. (1994a). *Clinical reasoning: Forms of inquiry in a therapeutic practice.* Philadelphia, PA: F. A. Davis.

Mattingly, C., & Fleming, M. (1994b). Interactive reasoning: Collaborating with the person. In C. Mattingly & M. H. Fleming (Eds.), *Clinical reasoning: Forms of inquiry in a therapeutic practice* (pp. 178-196). Philadelphia, PA: F. A. Davis.

McKeown, L. P., Porter-Armstrong, A., & Baxter, G. D. (2004). Caregivers of people with multiple sclerosis: Experiences of support. *Multiple Sclerosis, 10,* 219-230.

Miller, E., & Kuhaneck, H. (2008). Children's perceptions of play experiences and play preferences: A qualitative study. *American Journal of Occupational Therapy, 62,* 407-415.

Mitchell, J. M., & Kemp, B. J. (2000). Quality of life in assisted living homes: A multidimensional analysis. *Journal of Gerontology: Psychological Sciences, 55B,* P117-P127.

Myers, D. G. (2000). *The American paradox.* New Haven, MA: Yale University Press.

Naisbitt, J. (1982). *Megatrends: Ten directions transforming our lives.* New York, NY: Warner Books, Inc.

Palmer, P. J. (1987). Community, conflict, and ways of knowing. *Chance, 19,* 20-25.

Peloquin, S. M. (1993). The depersonalization of patients: A profile gleaned from narratives. *American Journal of Occupational Therapy, 47,* 830-837.

Peloquin, S. M. (1995). The fullness of empathy: Reflections and illustrations. *American Journal of Occupational Therapy, 49,* 24-31.

Peloquin, S. M. (2002). Confluence: Moving toward affective strength. *American Journal of Occupational Therapy, 56,* 69-77.

Primeau, L. A. (2000). Household work: When gender ideologies and practice interact. *Journal of Occupational Science, 7,* 118-127.

Primeau, L. A. (2003). Reflections on self in qualitative research: Stories of family. *American Journal of Occupational Therapy, 57,* 9-16.

Putnam, R. D. (2000). *Bowling alone: The collapse and revival of American community.* New York, NY: Simon & Schuster.

Rosa, S., & Hasselkus, B. R. (1996). Connecting with patients: The personal experience of professional helping. *Occupational Therapy Journal of Research, 16,* 245-260.

Rosa, S., & Hasselkus, B. R. (2005). Finding common ground with patients: The centrality of compatibility. *American Journal of Occupational Therapy, 59,* 198-208.

Rosengren, A., Orth-Gomer, K., Wedel, H., & Wilhelmsen, L. (1993). Stressful life events, social supports, and mortality in men born in 1933. *British Medical Journal, 307,* 1102-1105.

Sarton, M. (1973). *Journal of a solitude.* New York, NY: Norton.

Sarton, M. (1980). *Recovering: A journal.* New York, NY: Norton.

Schön, D. A. (1983). *The reflective practitioner: How professionals think in action.* New York, NY: Basic Books.

Ståhl, T., Rütten, A., Nutbeam, D., Bauman, A., Kannas, L., Abel, T., ... (2001). The importance of the social environment for physically active lifestyle—Results from an international study. *Social Science & Medicine, 52,* 1-10.

Stewart, K. B., & Meyer, L. (2004). Brief report: Parent-child interactions and everyday routines in young children with failure to thrive. *American Journal of Occupational Therapy, 58,* 342-346.

Sugisawa, H., Liang, J., & Liu, X. (1994). Social networks, social support, and mortality among older people in Japan. *Journal of Gerontology, 49,* S3-S13.

Taylor, R. R., Lee, S. W., Kielhofner, G., & Ketkar, M. (2009). Therapeutic use of self: A nation-wide survey of practitioners' attitudes and experiences. *American Journal of Occupational Therapy, 63,* 198-207.

Townsend, A., Langille, L., & Ripley, D. (2003). Professional tensions in client-centered practice: Using institutional ethnography to generate understanding and transformation. *American Journal of Occupational Therapy, 57,* 17-28.

Waitzkin, H. (1991). *The politics of medical encounters.* New Haven, CT: Yale University Press.

Ward, R. A. (1984). *The aging experience: An introduction to social gerontology.* New York, NY: Harper & Row.

Watson, R. (2004). A population approach to transformation. In R. Watson & L. Swartz (Eds.), *Transformation through occupation* (pp. 51-65). London, UK: Whurr Pub.

Whiteford, G. (2007). Artistry of the everyday: Connection, continuity and context. *Journal of Occupational Science, 14,* 77-81.

Wilcock, A. A. (1998). Reflections on doing, being and becoming. *Canadian Journal of Occupational Therapy, 65,* 248-256.

Wilcock, A. A. (2006). *An occupational perspective of health* (2nd ed.). Thorofare, NJ: SLACK Incorporated.

Zemke, R., & Clark, F. (1996). Co-occupation of mothers and children. In R. Zemke & F. Clark (Eds.), *Occupational science: The evolving discipline* (pp. 213-215). Philadelphia, PA: F. A. Davis.

# CHAPTER 7

# DISABILITY AND OCCUPATION

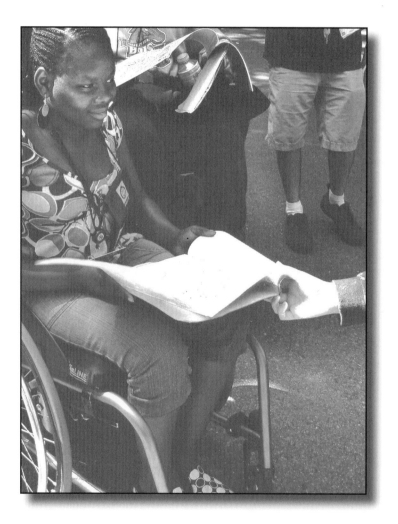

Disability scholars argue that impairment should be understood not as a personal lack or limitation, but as a unique way of being situated in the world.

Kielhofner (2005, p. 490)

In her personal journal, written in the ninth decade of her life, psychologist Florida Scott-Maxwell wrote that the basic task of daily life is to maintain the delicate balance between being "all right" and being overcome by the infirmities of old age; "The crucial task of age is balance, a veritable tightrope of balance; keeping just well enough, just brave enough, just gay and interested and starkly honest enough to remain a sentient human being" (1968, p. 36).

I think this tightrope of balance is a crucial task at all stages of life. When we are ill, we can accept the disability temporarily, but with each passing day, we get more and more impatient for the expected return to health. I remember walking around my house one morning, several years ago, in an absolute weeping rage because of the appearance of yet another migraine headache. Until I finally got the headaches under control, my life felt totally out of balance; *disability* ruled over *ability* with a heavy hand. The migraine sufferer, the child with a skinned knee, the older person who is bruised from a fall, the teenager with acne, the college student with mononucleosis—all are waiting and hoping for the balance of their lives to be restored, and all are expecting that balance *will* be restored.

So, too, is the tightrope of balance the crucial task in those circumstances when the disability is not temporary or fully remediable. When a baby is born with a disability, the parents find themselves torn by the wrenching *im*balance represented by the disability; they are living with the paradox of loving the baby—disability and all—at the same time that they continue to hope that the disability is temporary, that it will one day be gone, that the balance in their lives and in the baby's life will be restored (Larson, 1998; Layne, 1996). The person who has experienced a stroke, the daughter who is caring for her mother who has dementia, the young man who has a spinal cord injury—these people, too, are seeking balance in their lives, balance between ability and disability, hoping against all odds that a sense of balance *will* someday be regained.

Such is the power of the concept "disability." Disability is something that we do not want in our lives. Frank (2000) referred to this strong dictum about disability as our deeply ingrained "cultural view that disability is essentially undesirable" (p. 49). In their article on stigma and disability, Shuttleworth and Kasnitz (2004) made the statement that "… people with various chronic illnesses and impairments in different societies can often be stigmatized, that is, marked as different by others and socially devalued because of this difference" (p. 146). These authors stated further that, perhaps especially in the consumerist society of the United States, "the body beautiful is a lifestyle orientation that harbors an implicit moral reading of illness and impairment-disability" (p. 151). The body beautiful ideal is one of the social forces that creates stigmatization and devaluing associated with physical disability. We can tolerate disability temporarily, but we have a need to maintain the hope that the situation will change, that, in time, the balance will be restored, that *ability,* not disability, will govern our lives.

Hasselkus, B. R.
*The Meaning of Everyday Occupation, Second Edition* (pp. 125-142).
© 2011 SLACK Incorporated

# THE FACES OF DISABILITY

In the mid-twentieth century, to be disabled was defined as being incapable, incapacitated, in a state of incompetence in the physical, intellectual, or moral sense (Webster's New Collegiate Dictionary, 1956). Later in the century, the World Health Organization (1980) issued the first *International Classification of Impairment, Disability and Handicap* (ICIDH), using the word *disability* to stand for limitations in personal activities; the change from the earlier definition represented a shift away from the previous focus on incompetence per se toward a focus on the functional limitations that are the *result* of the incompetence. In the most recent version, the document title has been changed to *International Classification of Functioning, Disability and Health* (ICF; WHO, 2009); disability has been cast as a "universal human experience," the natural outcome of daily interactions between a person's bodily structure and function and his or her personal activities and participation in society. As stated in the introduction to the document on the Web site, the ICF "places all health conditions on an equal footing ... [it] takes into account the social aspects of disability and does not see disability only as a 'medical' or 'biological' dysfunction."

Clearly, the definition has moved toward disability as a socially defined phenomenon. Nevertheless, the ICF document with its classifications continues to be critiqued by scholars in disabilities studies, as well as by some in the field of occupational therapy (Hemmingsson & Jonsson, 2005; Wade & Halligan, 2003). A comprehensive definition of participation in society, one that reaches beyond observed performance, is held to be missing, as are the subjective experiences of meaning, autonomy, and self-determination (Hemmingsson & Jonsson). Further, recognition that different kinds of societal participation and environmental influences may be involved in even a single life situation is absent, yielding a one-dimensional view that is felt to ignore the complex reality of participation in life situations.

## Disability as a "Normal" Part of Life

In their study of the experience of cancer illness, Little, Jordens, Paul, Montgomery, and Philipson (1998) reflected on our history of a century ago, when illness and disability were accepted as simply part of the risks of the unpredictable life trajectory that human beings experienced: "Illness was simply part of the profile of risk. ... If one survived [an illness], one returned to living as before as best one could, surrounded by the same risk profile. Illness was an episode in 'normal' life" (p. 1492). In the ICF (WHO, 2009), as described above, an attempt has been made to return again to an image of disability as a universal phenomenon; in this view, disability occurs as a natural consequence of ordinary daily life—of the continuous interactions between our minds and bodies and the social and physical world around us.

In modern times, this view of disability as part of normal living has come to be associated with the concepts of holistic health (McColl, 1994; McKee, 1988). In a holistic view, illness and disability are understood as normal experiences of life; further, they are seen as opportunities for personal growth and development, occasions to achieve higher levels of "self-awareness and integration with the environment" (McColl, p. 72). Health is defined as "the experience of equilibrium and integration within oneself and one's environment" (McColl, p. 74). Through illness and disability, as through all life experiences, one can come to know one's self and one's world better.

The field of disabilities studies, emerging in the 1970s and 1980s, is in sync with many of the beliefs and practices of holistic health (Kielhofner, 2005). One goal of scholars in disabilities studies is to rethink disability so that it is understood "not as a personal lack or limitation, but as a unique way of being in the world ... impairments should not be defined in terms of how they differ from what is average or normal, but on their own terms as forms of human embodiment ... impairment is a natural part of human diversity" (Kielhofner, p. 490). The second goal of the disabilities studies movement is to give voice to disabled persons in ongoing discussions about the nature of disability. Incorporating this authentic voice into the conversation helps foster a self-definition of disability among disabled people, leading to more of a sense of ownership, positive identity and disability pride for people with disabilities. Both goals in disabilities studies are felt to be vitally important to shifting disability from a medical issue to a civil rights issue.

## Disability as an Adversary

The view of disability as a natural phenomenon of life is different from the biomedical view of disability as an abnormality of life. In the biomedical view, illness and disability are not part of ordinary life; they are phenomena to be eradicated or prevented or overcome (Jette, 1999). In the words of Little et al. (1998), with the rise of

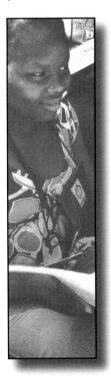

the biomedical dominance in Western health care systems, illness has become a state of alienation: "Illness is an aberration to be engineered out of existence" (p. 1492).

Jette (1999) and his colleagues (Field & Jette, 2007; Lawrence & Jette, 1996; Verbrugge & Jette, 1994) represent the biomedical face of disability in which disability is viewed as an adversary to be conquered. This adversarial view of illness and disability resonates throughout Western culture and is reflected strongly in the language of health and health care; we speak of "declaring war" on cancer, of "wiping out" diseases such as smallpox and polio, of "conquering" disability. Sontag (1991) has written about the military metaphors we often use in talking and writing about illness, especially about cancer. In obituary after obituary, we read of people who died of cancer only after waging a "courageous battle"; the words seem not to be used simply as a way to describe someone's final days but more as a badge of honor to the spirit of the one who has died. To have put up a good fight speaks well for a person.

The rehabilitation movement of the 1940s and 1950s grew out of these biomedical beliefs about disability. Today, for a person with a disability to have "rehabilitation potential" means that the person has the stamina and fortitude to withstand a rigorous schedule of daily therapy; further, it means that the person is motivated to work hard for long hours to *overcome* as much of his or her disabling condition as is humanly possible, to fight the good fight. The origins of the professions of occupational therapy, speech therapy, and physical therapy are imbedded in this rehabilitation ideology.

A critic might say that the biomedical view of disability is one that medicalizes the life of a person, framing and defining that life within medical boundaries that demand the mobilization of energies to conquer the disability and its consequent limitations. Alternatively, the holistic health view that illness and disability are natural phenomena of life invested with opportunities of their own is apt to be criticized for promoting passivity and a debilitating attitude of resignation.

Thus, we have two starkly different faces of disability. Both the biomedical and holistic views recognize functional differences and changes as part of the definition of disability, but they differ in terms of their philosophies of response to those changes. In the biomedical view, the crucial life task of achieving balance is approached by ridding oneself of the disability and its attendant limitations; balance is regained by expunging the aberration in order to get back to what life was like before or to what life is typically like for others. In the holistic view, we accomplish balance by accepting and living life within the boundaries of the disability, and by seeing, within functional changes, not an enemy to be conquered but, rather, different opportunities for growth and development.

## *Victory and Defeat*

I am not trying to argue that one face of disability is good and the other is bad. In her journal written late in life, Scott-Maxwell (1968) eloquently illustrated both views of disability. In the very first sentence of her book, she spoke of the dual nature of aging; that is, both the debility and the growth represented in growing old. She started her journal by stating, "We who are old know that age is more than a disability. It is an intense and varied experience, almost beyond our capacity at times, but something to be carried high. If it is a long defeat it is also a victory, meaningful for the initiates of time, if not for those who have come less far" (p. 5). Here is an expression of the experience of equilibrium and integration within oneself, found in the defeat as well as in the victory wrought by aging and disability. The "crucial task" of finding the balance between ability and disability is evident.

At one point in her journal, Scott-Maxwell (1968) focused on acute illnesses. She described having lived with major pain for some time, and eventually taking her doctor's advice and undergoing gall bladder surgery. She rejoiced in her newfound life afterwards: "I have life before me, better health, and less pain, less pain; the biggest pain gone for good, only bits of chronic pain left. … Not to have pain, even my degree of pain, which was always bearable, is a constant elation which will always be part of me" (p. 89). We can sense victory over disability in these words, a reclaiming of life more as it was "before," and a new balance in life that is grounds for elation, with "the biggest pain gone for good." Scott-Maxwell would probably say that some forms of disability *can* and *should* be eradicated and overcome.

Perhaps not surprisingly, some of the great philosophers of all time wrestled with these same issues concerning the nature of illness and health. Is illness simply one more necessary but normal aspect of life to be lived, or is illness an unnatural part of life, to be avoided or overcome? The 16th-century French philosopher Montaigne shared his thoughts on the natural balance of advantages and adversities in life as follows:

> Our life is composed, as is the harmony of the World, of contrary things; so of divers tunes, some pleasant, some harsh, some sharpe, some flat, some low, and some high. What would that Musition [musician] say that should love but some one of them? He ought to know how to use them severally and how to entermingle them. So should we both of goods and evils which are consubstantiall to our life. Our being cannot subsist without this commixture, whereto one side is no lesse necessary than the other. (Mendel, 1939, p. 145)

In de Botton's (2000) book on *The Consolations of Philosophy*, the author discussed Montaigne and five other great philosophers of all time. de Botton said that to Montaigne and others, "Fulfillment was to be reached not by avoiding pain, but by recognizing its role as a natural, inevitable step on the way to reaching anything good" (2000, p. 210). Or, as Montaigne said, "... one side is no lesse necessary than the other." Alternatively, Schopenhauer, a 20th-century German philosopher, strongly counseled that human beings should strive to avoid pain and live quietly, the opposite of Montaigne's urgings (de Botton).

I include these references to the great philosophers to alert the reader to the fact that the faces of disability are not simply contemporary issues, derived from contemporary society and contemporary thinking. These are, instead, issues that belong to the ages and that address one of the core meanings of life itself. Is disability friend or foe? Is it to be lived *with* or fought against? Is it to be accepted or overcome? It seems likely that disability is both friend *and* foe; the trick is to accept it as both but to somehow distinguish the aspects to be lived with from those that can and need to be defeated.

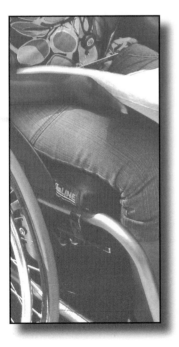

# OCCUPATION AS DISABILITY EXPERIENCE

Most people experience acute health problems of one type or another sometime in their lifetimes. During such a health crisis, the lives of all who are closely connected to the situation are affected; daily occupations are dramatically rearranged in deference to the needs of the moment—the crisis rules. In other words, during acute illness, people's everyday routines and activities—their occupations—are defined by the illness and disability. The more serious the illness, the more we accept the need to halt our usual day's occupations in order to focus our time and attention on the responsibilities that are defined and demanded by biomedical concerns.

## The Authority of Medical Crisis

The upheaval of everyday life that is the consequence of acute medical crises is vividly evident in the autobiographical paper by Linda Layne (1996) in which she describes her experience as the mother of a newborn premature baby being cared for on a neonatal infant care unit (NICU). She tells her story in day-by-day accounts; each episode is packed with the events and decisions surrounding the health and care of her newborn son, Jasper, on the NICU. She and her husband found themselves completely absorbed in the terrifying ups and downs ("a real roller coaster"; p. 633) of Jasper's condition. They learned about and watched for the subtle markers of positive progress such as the move from open warming tray to isolette, to crib; from an external heating system to a blanket; from intravenous feedings to nasogastric tube to oral feeds; from red preemie nipples to the beige, full-term nipples; and from breathing tube to nasal tube to room air.

During the health crisis, this family's absorption in Jasper's health seemed to be nearly complete; almost all other aspects of ordinary daily life were put aside and the medical crisis ruled over their lives. But over time, the daily occupations of Linda Layne and her family became less and less defined by medical needs and disability. In a one-paragraph Epilogue to the article, Layne (1996) relents from the consuming focus on the daily occupations of the NICU to recount the "happy" ending of Jasper's story—that by 2 years of age, he was bright and cheerful, loved "books, anything with wheels, and roughhousing with his older brother" (p. 642). By this point in time, the developmental pediatrician had assured them that "'disability' would be an optional term for Jasper" (p. 642); the message was that, ultimately, their lives might *not* be a disability experience after all.

## Occupational Therapy Defined by Disability

Much of the practice of occupational therapy is strongly defined by disability. For many of us, our practice settings, the reimbursement system under which we work, our referral systems, our educational curriculums, many of our interest groups, all reflect the medical aspects of our profession. In a practice defined by disability, the focus is on the remedial and recovery potential of occupation as defined by the illness.

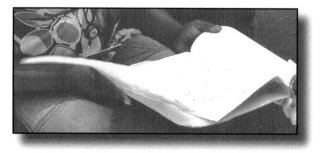

Literature that reflects the face of occupation as a disability experience is that which focuses on the effects of pathology and disease on occupation.

Typical of this literature is the study by Dighe, Aparasu, and Rappaport (1997) in which the relationship between activity limitations and survival in individuals who have experienced a stroke was examined. In another example, authors conducted a survey of assessment tools designed specifically to test driving skills of people with traumatic brain injuries (Classen, et al., 2009). Pfeiffer, Kinnealey, Reed, and Herzberg (2005) studied sensory modulation and affective disorders in children and adolescents with Asberger's disorder. Liu, McDowd, and Liu (2004) reported research on the relationship between visual inattention and daily life performance in people with dementia. A Canadian study in which the activity levels of children with and without asthma are compared is another example (Hessel, Sliwkanich, Michaelchuk, White, & Nguyen, 1996).

The focus on occupation as defined by disease, represented in the literature cited above, is a natural byproduct of the medical domain. In Rogers and Masagatani's (1982) early work on clinical reasoning, the data clearly revealed the strong reliance of occupational therapists on medical diagnoses for assessment and treatment planning in physical disabilities settings. Occupational therapy that is based on the belief that occupation can influence medical remediation and recovery from disease or injury or congenital disorder quite naturally focuses treatment on the etiological level of the condition; occupational therapy for clients after hip replacement, stroke, and traumatic brain injury are obvious examples. Occupational therapy for infants and children is often guided by the pathology of the underlying disorder as it interacts with a child's developmental requirements. Our emerging literature on occupational therapy in neo-natal care (Bartlett & Piper, 1993; Case-Smith, Butcher, & Reed, 1998) and our rather vast literature on occupational therapy for children with sensory integrative disorders are examples. This is not to say that in these situations occupational therapists focus *only* on the biomedical foundations of occupation; rather, I am pointing out that under circumstances such as these, the focus of the therapy is, at least initially, heavily on the underlying pathology.

When we find ourselves as occupational therapy practitioners in biomedical settings, with a strong practice focus on the eradication or amelioration of disease and disability, we are, ipso facto, aligned with the view that disease and disability are aberrations of life that need to be fought and conquered. Rewards for the therapist in this situation occur when he or she feels that the effects of an underlying pathological condition on daily occupation have been diminished by the occupational therapy process, and that a client has become less disabled and more competent for living life because of our treatment.

Remember the therapist's story (Chapter 5) of the 16-year-old boy who had sustained a spinal cord injury in a diving accident; the therapist said:

> With the use of EMG biofeedback and everything else we were doing in therapy, just general ADLs and strengthening activities and isolated muscle strengthening … he's regained a lot of function in his hands, his arms; he's got a car now, he's independent in transfers back and forth from the car. He had a job this summer at the pool. … He's back in the social swing of things and just really has come a long, long, long way (Hasselkus & Dickie, 1994, raw data).

The therapist's sense of accomplishment and satisfaction related to the changes brought about by medical rehabilitation is evident.

## The Loss of Humanness

The "down" side of practice in a biomedical setting occurs when a client becomes so strongly identified with a disease or disability in the eyes of a therapist as well as others that the humanness of the patient is diminished or lost (Latimer, 1999). Little et al. (1998), in their study of the experience of chronic illness and cancer, reported that one of the consistent concerns of the people with cancer who were interviewed was "a persisting identification as a cancer patient, regardless of the time since treatment and of the presence or absence of persistent or recurrent disease" (p. 1485).

Clinical routines and procedures objectify clients, placing them in what Lock (1993) called *marked categories* ("cancer patient"); loss of self and identity can be the result. Jasper, who was born at 30 weeks' gestation, was referred to by the NICU nurses as a "30-weeker." Linda became part of a group known by the nurses as "the moms." These labels served to objectify Jasper and Linda (i.e., to erase their individuality); at least these particular labels, however, were fairly innocuous and neutral in most regards. To be labeled "disabled," "an arthritic," "an amputee," or "an alcoholic," however, is to be ascribed a clinical identity that is far from neutral; medical identities often carry very negative meanings, perhaps especially those that are believed to be caused by personal behaviors such as identities associated with HIV/AIDS, alcoholism, lung cancer, or attempted suicide.

Perhaps it is obvious that the technology of rehabilitation and long term care can place people into marked categories. The typical accoutrements of rehabilitation and long-term care such as assistive devices, braces and splints, wheelchairs, and other technologies are like double-edged swords (Lupton & Seymour, 2000; Oliver, 1990; Roulstone, 1998; Scherer, 1993) because, although such pieces of equipment may contribute to increased mobility and independence, they also contribute to an identity of being disabled. Lupton and Seymour studied the ways in which technologies contribute to the meanings and experiences of the self with disabilities. Although the people who were interviewed in the study identified several technologies as highly beneficial to overcoming aspects of their disabilities, they also identified significant negative aspects of some of the same technologies, saying that they served to mark people with disabilities as "different" and acted as barriers to the presentation of their preferred selves.

These risks to identity and to self are inherent in the occupational therapy process when occupation is defined by disability. Cohen (1994) declared carers associated with biomedicine to be the greatest offenders in this regard. In biomedical settings, we care providers are vulnerable to seeing patients *as* their diagnoses and to categorizing clients and patients by their illnesses and disabilities. The therapist described earlier was pleased and proud that the 16-year-old fellow with whom she worked in rehabilitation had begun to reestablish himself in the community with his regained mobility and a new job. With this description of independence and engagement in the community, it does not seem like the therapist was placing this adolescent into a marked category; the therapist does not sound as though she was seeing the 16-year-old *as* his diagnosis. And yet, at the beginning of her story, in her very first reference to the young man, she referred to him as "a 16-year-old quadriplegic from a diving accident—C6 or 7, incomplete." Such is the language of medical care and, as we all know, the language we use reflects the reality that we live.

# DISABILITY AS OCCUPATIONAL EXPERIENCE

During the last two decades of the 20th century, we witnessed an expansion in the occupational therapy profession toward defining illness and wellness as phenomena that are *occupationally experienced* as well as physiologically experienced. Starting with Kielhofner's (1981) early work on understanding the daily life experiences of adults with mental retardation from an occupational perspective, our literature has gradually evolved to include works that focus first on the nature and experience of occupation and secondarily on an illness context. A few of the many examples of this focus on occupation can be readily seen in such titles as: "Returning to School After a Spinal Cord Injury: Perspectives From Four Adolescents" (Mulcahey, 1992); "Contextual Factors and Participation in Employment for People With Serious Mental Illness" (Henry & Lucca, 2002); "The Meaning of Work After Acquired Brain Injury" (Johansson & Tham, 2006); "Everyday Lives of People With Advanced Cancer: Activity, Time, Location, and Experience" (la Cour, Nordell, & Josephsson, 2009); and *Navigating in a Changing World: Experiences of Everyday Life From the Perspective of Persons With Cognitive Impairment or Dementia* (Öhman, 2007).

Disability is still strongly present in the literature but more often as a backdrop to the up-front emphasis on time use, activity patterns, life roles, and occupational experiences. This shifting view obviously does not disregard the contribution of disease and pathology to the situation; it represents, however, an important reorientation to increasingly granting primacy to occupation rather than to illness.

If you have read any of the many works written by people who are experiencing disability, you already know that people define their disabilities by their occupations (see Bayley, 1999; Frank, 2000; Sarton, 1988; Scott-Maxwell, 1968). Both long-term chronic illness and short-term recovery are described in occupational terms. Only in situations of acute illness do people and their lives seem to be defined by disease.

## *Health as the Return to Familiar Routines*

The natural tendency of people to define their illnesses and disabilities as occupational experiences is illustrated by Florida Scott-Maxwell's (1968) journal descriptions of her convalescence after her gall bladder surgery. In the first days after her surgery, Scott-Maxwell bowed to the biomedical aspects of the hospital experience, describing herself as "lost in pain and drugs" (p. 92). On the fourth day, she looked down and "saw the great wound healed for most of its length" (p. 93); this sign of healing seemed to release her from the body focus, and from then on she described her recovery in terms of what she could *do*. "At last I was allowed a bath in a tub, though with a nurse to direct my every move. ... I hopped from my bed and watered my flowers. … I got up, threw back the curtains, opened all four windows … and expanded into the blue sky. Or so my whole heart longed to do. I wanted to be out of my body, without limit, I was rejuvenated, young, I wanted a future" (pp. 94-95). By the fifth day after surgery, Scott-Maxwell was feeling so much better that she 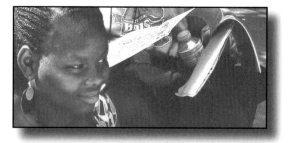 wrote, "More and more I belonged to myself" (p. 95). On the twelfth day, she felt so well that she took a walk by the sea; she wrote, "I felt so well that I thought it was the air that was curing me, for *now I did everything for myself, even making my bed*" (p. 96, emphasis added).

Scott-Maxwell used descriptions of everyday activities to convey her state of being once the acute stage of illness had passed; she defined her disability by occupation. The litany of gradually returning abilities and the occupations represented by those abilities offer us her record of recovery from surgery, until at last she is able to do "everything" for herself, even making her bed. Scott-Maxwell's story represents, to me, a portrayal of illness and disability as events that are occupationally experienced—that are defined by occupation.

In the past, I have offered the portrayal of the rehabilitation process as one of facilitating a gradual return to previous daily living routines (Hasselkus, 1994): "During rehabilitation, the individual seeks to maintain or re-establish habits and patterns of daily occupation that have gradually developed over many years" (p. 98). I likened this gradual return to previous daily patterns and routines to a process of convergence, adapted from social systems theory (Lennard & Bernstein, 1970). We might think of occupational therapy as a profession that is dedicated to facilitating the convergence process to help bring about the return over time of clients' self-responsibility and previous life patterns of occupation.

In an innovative expansion of convergence thinking, Gillen (2005) interviewed survivors of acute stroke, seeking to understand if they could name any positive consequences of the stroke experience. Many of the respondents described positive changes such as increased social relationships, personal growth, and increases in their health awareness. For the majority of the participants in Gillen's study, rehabilitation resulted in more than a return to previous ways of life; rehabilitation also led to the development of new and valued interests and ways of being in the world.

Bloom's (2001) findings in his study of the quality of life of gay men during the course of HIV infection offer more evidence of the power and meaning of familiar everyday routines in people's lives. Using life story narratives gathered across two years of repeated interviews with each of 20 participants (five of the participants died by the end of the second year), Bloom generated several life themes, including one theme he called "average life" (p. 46). The average life theme, represented by the narratives of four men in the study, was a theme of contentment with "maintaining an everyday life that is uneventful, mundane, and 'boring'" (p. 46). One of the four men with this theme described his life as "routine and predictable" (p. 46); all four participants expressed the hope that their average, uneventful lives would continue indefinitely. In

Bloom's interpretation, this average life theme symbolized for the men in the study a kind of normalcy over the course of the illness and their lives; if daily life is uneventful and predictable, then life is near normal and full of familiarity, and the impact of the disease on one's identity and autonomy is within normal limits. "Being boring is seen as highly desirable" (p. 49) when compared to the potential life-disrupting events associated with illness crises and complications.

To think of "boring" and "uneventful" as potentially such strong and positive contributors to the quality of life of people in *any* situation or context is an eye-opener. For the four men with HIV infection in Bloom's (2001) study, the enactment of the mundane routines of daily life enabled them to feel like they were still part of the mainstream of their society, and that they were still who they had always been. They were not *different*; they still fit in. This concept of disability as "difference," and of the meaning of habits and routines in everyday occupation, are addressed more fully in Chapter 4.

The power of habits, routines, and rituals to contribute to our sense of well-being and to our sense of belonging in the larger culture—to be insiders, not outsiders—is compelling to think about. As Clark (2000) has said, these daily, repetitive behaviors contribute to the construction of our identity and to our quality of life.

## Ill Health as the Loss of Familiar Occupations

Just as health may be thought of as the ability to carry out one's usual daily occupations, so *ill* health may be thought of as the loss of the ability to carry out familiar occupations. In Mitch Albom's (1997) beautifully crafted book about his former professor, Morrie, written as the professor lived out the last months before his death from amyotrophic lateral sclerosis, the markers of change across the weekly visits were clearly occupational. The significance of those markers to both Mitch and to Morrie was undeniable. What Morrie had anticipated with the most dread, and what symbolized the extremis of the illness situation to him, was losing the ability to "wipe his behind." After his seventh weekly visit, Albom wrote:

> Morrie lost his battle. Someone was now wiping his behind. ... It took some getting used to, Morrie admitted, because it was, in a way, complete surrender to the disease. The most personal and basic things had now been taken from him—going to the bathroom, wiping his nose, washing his private parts. With the exception of breathing and swallowing his food, he was dependent on others for nearly everything. (p. 115)

In contrast to Scott-Maxwell (1968) who, in her recovery, rejoiced in getting "out of my body," Morrie was becoming more and more "owned" by his body and the disease. The movement in opposite directions is telling—Scott-Maxwell *out of her body* and *toward* occupation, and Morrie further and further *into his body* and more and more *distanced from* occupation.

In occupational therapy, we try to accompany people on their journeys, whether they are journeys of prevention and wellness, or of acute illness, congenital disorder, chronic illness and disability, or terminal illness, and whether they are journeys toward occupation or away from occupation. In progressive illnesses or in dying, such as with Morrie, we try to help people hold onto some semblance of their occupational definition of themselves and their days as they journey more and more into the disability and their bodies (Jacques & Hasselkus, 2004). In recovery, as with Scott-Maxwell, we try to promote convergence to help people regain the occupational definition of their lives. For those with a congenital disorder, such as Jasper, we try to enable them to achieve an occupational definition of their lives rather than a definition by disability; for Jasper's mother, we try to enable her to live again a life of wellness and ordinary everyday occupation. In chronic disability, as with the 16-year-old youth with a spinal cord injury, we try to promote adaptation and acceptance of a new occupational definition of life.

## Occupational Experiences as Health Promoting

In recent years, a kind of broadening of our basic images of ourselves as occupational therapists and as occupational science researchers has occurred. This broadened view continues to include the medical model and its accompanying emphasis on disease and illness, but it has also expanded into new ideas for research and practice related to occupation in the lives of all people, with and without disabilities.

Clark et al. (1997; see also Jackson, Carlson, Mandel, Zemke, & Clark, 1998; Jackson et al., 2009), in their study of lifestyle redesign among well-elderly people in a Los Angeles suburb, provided an example in our literature of the study of occupation without an illness or disability context. The occupational therapy intervention in this randomized controlled clinical trials study was designed to help well-elderly participants appreciate the importance of meaningful occupation in their lives and to share specific knowledge about how to select and take part in occupations so as to achieve a healthy and satisfying lifestyle. Involvement in the research increased the well-elderly participants' awareness of the importance of meaningful and healthful daily routines in the context of their lives. The occupational definitions of their daily lives gained prominence and focus; daily routines and activities became conscious occupational experiences. In Scott-Maxwell's (1968) words, balance—the crucial task of age—had been attended to and strengthened.

## BEING THE BRIDGE

Those of us in occupational therapy are in some ways in a tough spot; we somehow want to have our feet in both camps; that is, to be part of the medical team but also to be part of the non-medical life context of the people with whom we work. We recognize and believe in the power of occupation to reflect who people are and to tell us the state of people's health. In reality, we are positioned like a bridge, spanning and linking the world of medical health with the world of everyday life. We are, perhaps, the sturdiest and most accessible bridge between these two worlds. Maybe *being the bridge* is our unique role in community and medical care.

In occupational therapy, we juggle biomedical and holistic responses to disability; we attempt to function in both the medical world of recovery and rehabilitation *and* in the world of living with disability as a natural experience of life. Mattingly (1994a) has referred to this dual nature of occupational therapy as a "two-body practice" (p. 64), meaning that therapists address both the biomedical bodies and the phenomenological or experiential bodies of the people with whom they work. Wilcock (2006) refers to this view of health that melds together the biological and the experiential as an occupational perspective of health.

## A Difficult Balancing Act

Maintaining a balance between the biomedical and phenomenological practices is a delicate challenge; this balancing act may be *our* crucial task. Creating or maintaining a balance may be especially difficult in long-term care settings such as public schools and nursing homes (Hasselkus, Dickie, & Gregory, 1997; Niehues, Bundy, Mattingly, & Lawlor, 1991). Magasi and Hammel (2009) provide a stunning example of this balancing act in their study of the experiences of women with disabilities in long-term care. To these women, life in the nursing home was characterized by many losses including loss of choice, control, occupational engagement, and social participation. The authors concluded that occupational therapists have a responsibility to ensure that residents live in the least restrictive environments possible, and that "long-term-care referral practices, advocacy-based interventions, and partnership with the disability community" become part of our practice (p. 35). Clearly, the subjective and experiential aspects of disability are at the core in this study, and the implications reach far beyond the individual client and her biomedical needs to the *system* of long-term care.

A balance is also a challenge in settings such as rehabilitation centers (Chang & Hasselkus, 1998). In rehabilitation, a trajectory of expected physiological improvement is strongly present in the early stages of the process. An initial period of remediation, however, may at some point in time end in a plateau, a stage of recovery when "the client has reached a relatively stable and unchanging state" (Chang & Hasselkus, 1998, p. 635). For example, in rehabilitation for clients following stroke, therapists focus during the early stage of treatment on the physiological and biomechanical functions of "the arm and hand" (p. 631); at this stage, balance in life seems to be defined by both therapists and patients as regaining pre-stroke levels of motor control and movement in the body parts. Once a plateau of recovery has been reached, therapists turn their attention (sometimes reluctantly) to the clients' adaptation strategies and functional compensations, i.e., toward a new kind of balance in life, a balance that encompasses living with the stroke and its residual effects. At this often difficult turning point in therapy, not only must the therapist shift his or her own perspective and expectations, but the therapist most likely has to help the client change perspectives as well, for the client, too, will have been focused on the biomedical improvement of the physical body; to relinquish hopes and expectations for a full "recovery" and to settle, instead, for finding fulfillment in strategies of adaptation and a modified lifestyle is bound to be a difficult proposition.

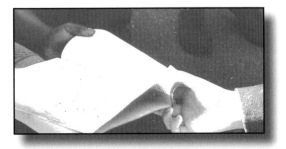

In occupational therapy, we are often faced with this difficult task of embodying both faces of disability, and with the challenge of guiding clients in the journey from one to the other. We operate in an arena of paradoxes since we typically persuade a client to focus on the medical aspects of his or her situation in the early stages of therapy in order to enhance the chances of ultimately being able to *not* focus on the medical aspects. To the client and family, this shift in emphasis may seem like an inconsistency in the therapy, yet the underlying process and rationale may represent best practice in rehabilitation. The early stages of therapy reflect occupation as a disability experience; the later stages represent disability as an occupational experience.

The current programs of training for occupational therapy personnel seem to lead to expectations in practice for a progressive trajectory of improved function, regained independence, and maintenance of, or return to, previous lifestyles (Becker & Kaufman, 1995; Mattingly, 1994b). We are only more recently beginning to reconceptualize our practice to fit with situations in which a trajectory of "improvement" is not necessarily the backbone of occupational therapy, and goals of living *with* one's self and finding fulfillment *in* one's self—whatever the state of that self may be—are legitimate goals for therapy (Hasselkus, Dickie, & Gregory, 1997; Niehues, Bundy, Mattingly, & Lawlor, 1991). The shift to conceptualizing disability defined by occupation as well as occupation defined by disability reflects this expanding view of occupational therapy practice.

# REFERENCES

Albom, M. (1997). *Tuesdays with Morrie: An old man, a young man, and life's greatest lesson.* New York, NY: Doubleday.

Bartlett, D., & Piper, M. D. (1993). Neuromotor development of preterm infants through the first year of life: Implications for physical and occupational therapists. *Physical & Occupational Therapy in Pediatrics, 12*(4), 37-55.

Bayley, J. (1999). *Elegy for Iris.* New York, NY: Picador USA.

Becker, G., & Kaufman, S. (1995). Managing an uncertain illness trajectory in old age: Patients' and physicians' views of stroke. *Medical Anthropology Quarterly, 9,* 165-187.

Bloom, F. R. (2001). "New beginnings": A case study in gay men's changing perceptions of quality of life during the course of HIV infection. *Medical Anthropology Quarterly, 15,* 38-57.

Case-Smith, J., Butcher, L., & Reed, D. (1998). Parents' report of sensory responsiveness and temperament in preterm infants. *American Journal of Occupational Therapy, 52,* 547-555.

Chang, L.-H., & Hasselkus, B. R. (1998). Occupational therapists' expectations in rehabilitation following stroke: Sources of satisfaction and dissatisfaction. *American Journal of Occupational Therapy, 52,* 629-637.

Clark, F., Azen, S. P., Zemke, R., Jackson, J., Carlson, M., Mandel, D., ... Lipson, L. (1997). Occupational therapy for independent-living older adults. *Journal of the American Medical Association, 278,* 1321-1326.

Clark, F. A. (2000). The concepts of habit and routine: A preliminary theoretical synthesis. *Occupational Therapy Journal of Research, 20*(Suppl.), 123S-137S.

Classen, S., Levy, C., McCarthy, D., Mann, W. C., Lanford, D., & Ward-Ebbs, J.K. (2009). Traumatic brain injury and driving assessment: An evidence-based literature review. *American Journal of Occupational Therapy, 63,* 580-591.

Cohen, A. (1994). *Self-consciousness: An alternative anthropology of identity*. London, UK: Routledge.

de Botton, A. (2000). *The consolations of philosophy*. New York, NY: Pantheon Books.

Dighe, M. S., Aparasu, R. R., & Rappaport, H. M. (1997). Factors predicting survival, changes in activity limitations, and disability in a geriatric post-stroke population. *The Gerontologist, 37*, 483-489.

Field, M. J., & Jette, A. (Eds.). (2007). *The future of disability in America*. Washington, DC: The National Academies Press.

Frank, G. (2000). *Venus on wheels: Two decades of dialogue on disability, biography, and being female in America*. Berkeley: University of California Press.

Gillen, G., (2005). Brief report—Positive consequences of surviving a stroke. *American Journal of Occupational Therapy, 59*, 346-350.

Hasselkus, B. R. (1994). From hospital to home: Family-professional relationships in geriatric rehabilitation. *Gerontology & Geriatric Education, 15*(1), 91-100.

Hasselkus, B. R., & Dickie, V. A. (1994). Doing occupational therapy: Dimensions of satisfaction and dissatisfaction. *American Journal of Occupational Therapy, 48*, 145-154.

Hasselkus, B. R., Dickie, V. A., & Gregory, C. (1997). Geriatric occupational therapy: The uncertain ideology of long-term care. *American Journal of Occupational Therapy, 51*, 132-139.

Hemmingsson, H., & Jonsson, H. (2005). An occupational perspective on the concept of participation in the International Classification of Functioning, Disability and Health—some critical remarks. *American Journal of Occupational Therapy, 59*, 569-576.

Henry, A. D., & Lucca, A. M. (2002). Contextual factors and participation in employment for people with serious mental illness. *Occupational Therapy Journal of Research, 22*(Suppl.), 835-845.

Hessel, P. A., Sliwkanich, T., Michaelchuk, D., White, H., & Nguyen, T.-H. (1996). Asthma and limitation of activities in Fort Saskatchewan, Alberta. *Canadian Journal of Public Health , 87*, 397-400.

Jackson, J., Carlson, M., Mandel, D., Zemke, R., & Clark, F. (1998). Occupation in lifestyle redesign: The well elderly study occupational therapy program. *American Journal of Occupational Therapy, 52*, 326-336.

Jackson, J. M., Mandel, D., Blanchard, J., Carlson, M. E., Cherry, B. J., Azen, S. P., ... (2009). Confronting challenges in intervention research with ethnically diverse older adults: The USC well elderly II trial. *Clinical Trials, 6*, 90-101.

Jacques, N., & Hasselkus, B. R. (2004). The nature of occupation surrounding dying and death. *OTJR: Occupation, Participation and Health, 24*, 44-53.

Jette, A. (1999). Disentangling the process of disablement. *Social Science & Medicine, 48*, 471-472.

Johansson, U., & Tham, K. (2006). The meaning of work after acquired brain injury. *American Journal of Occupational Therapy, 60*, 60-69.

Kielhofner, G. (1981). An ethnographic study of deinstitutionalized adults: Their community settings and daily life experiences. *Occupational Therapy Journal of Research, 1*, 125-142.

Kielhofner, G. (2005). Rethinking disability and what to do about it: Disability studies and its implications for occupational therapy. *American Journal of Occupational Therapy, 59*, 487-496.

la Cour, K., Nordell, K., & Josephsson, S. (2009). Everyday lives of people with advanced cancer: Activity, time, location, and experience. *OTJR: Occupation, Participation, and Health, 29*,154-162.

Larson, E. (1998). Reframing the meaning of disability to families: The embrace of paradox. *Social Science & Medicine, 47*, 865-875.

Latimer, J. (1999). The dark at the bottom of the stairs: Performance and participation of hospitalized older people. *Medical Anthropology Quarterly, 13,* 186-213.

Lawrence, R., & Jette, A. (1996). Disentangling the disablement process. *Journal of Gerontology: Social Sciences, 51B,* S173-S182.

Layne, L. L. (1996). "How's the baby doing?" Struggling with narratives of progress in a neonatal intensive care unit. *Medical Anthropology Quarterly, 10,* 624-656.

Lennard, H. L., & Bernstein, A. (1970). *Patterns in human interaction.* San Francisco, CA: Jossey-Bass.

Little, M., Jordens, C. F. C., Paul, K., Montgomery, K., & Philipson, B. (1998). Liminality: A major category of the experience of cancer illness. *Social Science & Medicine, 47,* 1485-1494.

Liu, C., McDowd, J., & Liu, K. (2004). Visuospatial inattention and daily life performance in people with Alzheimer's disease. *American Journal of Occupational Therapy, 58,* 202-210.

Lock, M. (1993). The politics of mid-life and menopause: Ideologies for the second sex in North America and Japan. In S. Lindenbaum & M. Lock (Eds.), *Knowledge, power and practice: The anthropology of medicine and everyday life* (pp. 330-363). Berkeley, CA: University of California Press.

Lupton, D., & Seymour, W. (2000). Technology, selfhood and physical disability. *Social Science & Medicine, 50,* 1851-1862.

Magasi, A., & Hammel, J. (2009). Women with disabilities' experiences in long-term care: A case for social justice. *American Journal of Occupational Therapy, 63,* 35-45.

Mattingly, C. (1994a). Occupational therapy as a two-body practice. In C. Mattingly, & M. Fleming (Eds.), *Clinical reasoning: Forms of inquiry in a therapeutic practice* (pp. 37-93). Philadelphia, PA: F. A. Davis.

Mattingly, C. (1994b). The concept of therapeutic "emplotment." *Social Science & Medicine, 38,* 811-822.

McColl, M. A. (1994). Holistic occupational therapy: Historical meaning and contemporary implications. *Canadian Journal of Occupational Therapy, 61,* 72-77.

McKee, J. (1988). Holistic health and the critique of Western medicine. *Social Science & Medicine, 26,* 775-784.

Mendel, A. O. (Ed.). (1939). *The living thoughts of Montaigne. Presented by Andre Gide.* Philadelphia, PA: David McKay.

Mulcahey, M. J. (1992). Returning to school after a spinal cord injury: Perspectives from four adolescents. *American Journal of Occupational Therapy, 46,* 305-312.

Niehues, A. N., Bundy, A. C., Mattingly, C. F., & Lawlor, M. C. (1991). Making a difference: Occupational therapy in the public schools. *Occupational Therapy Journal of Research, 11,* 195-212.

Öhman, A. (2007). *Navigating in a changing world: Experiences of everyday life from the perspective of persons with cognitive impairment or dementia.* Stockholm, Sweden: Karolinska Institutet.

Oliver, M. (1990). *The politics of disablement.* London, UK: Macmillan.

Pfeiffer, B., Kinnealey, M., Reed, C., & Herzberg, G. (2005). Sensory modulation and affective disorders in children and adolescents with Asberger's disorder. *American Journal of Occupational Therapy, 59,* 335-345.

Rogers, J., & Masagatani, G. (1982). Clinical reasoning of occupational therapists during the initial assessment of physically disabled patients. *Occupational Therapy Journal of Research, 2,* 195-219.

Roulstone, A. (1998). Researching a disabling society: The case of employment and new technology. In T. Shakespeare (Ed.), *The disability reader: Social science perspectives* (pp. 110-128). London, UK: Cassell.

Sarton, M. (1988). *After the stroke: A journal.* New York, NY: Norton.

Scherer, M. J. (1993). *Living in the state of stuck: How technology impacts the lives of people with disabilities.* Cambridge, MA: Brooldine Books.

Scott-Maxwell, F. (1968). *The measure of my days.* New York, NY: Alfred A. Knopf.

Shuttleworth, R. P., & Kasnitz, D. (2004). Stigma, community, ethnography: Joan Ablon's contribution to the anthropology of impairment-disability. *Medical Anthropology Quarterly, 18,* 139-161.

Sontag, S. (1991). *Illness as metaphor and AIDS and its metaphors.* Harmondsworth, UK: Penguin Books.

Verbrugge, L., & Jette, A. (1994). The disablement process. *Social Science & Medicine, 38,* 1-14.

Wade, D. T., & Halligan, P. (2003). New wine in old bottles: The WHO ICF as an explanatory model of human behavior. *Clinical Rehabilitation, 17,* 349-354.

*Webster's new collegiate dictionary.* (1956). Springfield, MA: G. & C. Merriam Co.

Wilcock, A. A. (2006). *An occupational perspective on health* (2nd ed.). Thorofare, NJ: SLACK Incorporated.

World Health Organization. (1980). *International classification of impairments, disabilities and handicaps.* Author.

World Health Organization. (2009). *International classification of functioning, disability and health.* Retrieved October 28, 2009 from www.who.int/classifications/icf/en/

CHAPTER 8

# OCCUPATION AS A SOURCE OF SPIRITUALITY

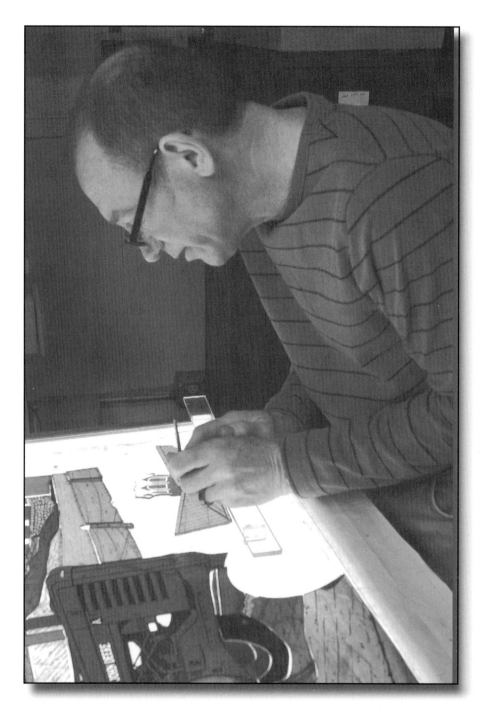

I believe that in the quiet, repetitive, hypnotic rhythms of creating craft, the inner being may emerge in all its quiet beauty.

Lydon (1997, p. 143)

In this chapter, I explore the concept of occupation as spiritual activity. This exploration is both from the standpoint of the potential for occupation to enrich spirituality—as is illustrated in the quotation from Susan Lydon's (1997) book on craft as a spiritual practice—and the potential for spirituality to enrich occupation. The meaning of spirituality is probed and literature on the concept of spiritual health is reviewed. The evolution of thinking within the profession is briefly presented as it relates to spirituality in everyday occupation and occupational therapy. Disagreement among therapists about the recent inclusion of spirituality in our publications and about the appropriateness or inappropriateness of spirituality in our practice is aired. The reader's own thinking on spirituality and occupation will hopefully be stirred.

## THIS THING CALLED SPIRITUALITY

In his book on the stages of faith, Fowler (1981) said that questions of spirituality "aim to help us get in touch with the dynamic, patterned process by which we find life meaningful" (p. 3). Further, "We require meaning. We need purpose and priorities, we must have some grasp on the big picture" (p. 4). In other words, spirituality is a dimension of living that helps us find coherence and meaning in our lives.

What is this thing called *spirituality*? A mere glance at the literature reveals the struggle that inevitably accompanies efforts to define this phenomenon of life (Hammell, 2003; McColl, 2003). Spirituality cannot be directly observed in the physical sense. We are not even at all sure what behaviors we might identify that *represent* this phenomenon. We have trouble finding the words to describe what we think we mean when we use the word spirituality. And yet, we probably all acknowledge the existence of some sort of spiritual nature in ourselves and in the lives of all human beings. As McFadden and Gerl (1990) stated, "The inability to articulate clearly the sense of spiritual integration should not be taken as a sign of its absence" (p. 37).

### Spirituality as an Inside Room

In her extraordinary first novel entitled *The Heart Is a Lonely Hunter*, Carson McCullers (1940) offers us a powerful image of spirituality. The lead character in the book is a 13-year-old girl named Mick Kelly. The story is set in a small Southern town, and the characters in the book represent a richly varied collection of human beings of various ages and stations in life. The novel is a deeply compelling narration of Mick's struggle with her impoverished lot in life juxtaposed with her intense personal search for beauty in her approaching adulthood. Her search for beauty can be likened to a spiritual journey as Mick seeks to come to know and to nurture her inner being.

Often in the evening, Mick's search for beauty takes her to another part of town where she sits in the dark, outside the open window of a certain house, and listens to the music being broadcast from the radio in the parlor inside. On one particular night, the radio programs had been "no good"; Mick has only been half listening and feeling like she was empty. Then she heard the announcer mention someone named Beethoven and a third symphony. As the music started:

Hasselkus, B. R.
*The Meaning of Everyday Occupation, Second Edition* (pp. 145-162).
© 2011 SLACK Incorporated

Mick raised her head and her fist went up to her throat. ... She could not listen good enough to hear it all. The music boiled inside her. Which? To hang
on to certain wonderful parts and think them over so that later she would
not forget—or should she let go and listen to each part that came without
thinking or trying to remember? Golly! The whole world was this music and
she could not listen hard enough. (McCullers, 1940, p. 100)

Later in the book, McCullers (1940) describes Mick's world as having "two places—
the inside room and the outside room" (p. 138). The outside room was full of school
and the family and the things that happen every day; music was part of the inside
room. "And the symphony. When she was by herself in this inside room, the music she
had heard that night after the party would come back to her. This symphony grew slow
like a big flower in her mind" (p. 138).

The metaphor of the inside room and the outside room is one way to think of spirituality. Perhaps it is in the inside room that the spirit of life resides, where passion and
significance take shape, where we are able to get in touch with the "dynamic, patterned process" talked about by Fowler (1981, p. 3). Perhaps, like Mick, most of our
dealings with other people and the rest of the world take place in the outside room,
and our experiences of interiority and conscious meaning are instances of our less
frequent habitation of the inside room.

## SPIRITUAL "HEALTH"

The term *spiritual health* has been used by some to describe an optimal state of
balance in life between the spiritual essence of one's inner being and the worldly connections of one's outer self. Chapman (1986) used the term *spiritual health* to describe
a person's state of being when engaged in an optimum level of searching for meaning
in life; too little interest in the search can lead to loneliness, alienation, and dissatisfaction, and excessive preoccupation can negatively affect family relationships, voca-
tional pursuits, and development of the self. It is optimal and healthful to balance the
energy devoted to the search for meaning with that devoted to more worldly pursuits.

Chapman's (1986) conceptualization of spirituality within a framework of health represents one of many such efforts found in the nursing and health promotion literature.
*Spiritual well-being, spiritual integrity,* and *spiritual health* are terms used to describe a
state of spiritual wholeness (Bellingham, Cohen, Jones, & Spaniol, 1989; Highfield &
Cason, 1983; Miller, 1985; Stoll, 1989). Alternatively, *spiritual distress* is a term used to
describe a pervasive disruption in a person's spiritual life (Heliker, 1992). The relationship between a health professional and a patient is characterized by some as a spiritual
relationship (Reed, 1992; Stiles, 1990). Spiritual beliefs and practices related to health,
attempts to measure spirituality, and goals for treatment planning and practice related
to spirituality have been proposed (Banks, 1980; Burkhardt, 1994; Chapman, 1987;
McFadden & Gerl, 1990; Pollner, 1989). Clearly, spirituality and health are intimately
related in the minds of many health and health care scholars.

Writers on spiritual health struggle to come up with tangible definitions and models of this intangible dimension of life. Bellingham et al. (1989) defined spiritual health as "the ability to live in the wholeness of life" (p. 18); they identified connectedness as the key to spiritual health—"connectedness to self, connectedness to others, and connectedness to a larger meaning or purpose" in life (p. 18). Sullivan (1993) extended this definition to include "one's personalized experience and identity pertaining to a sense of worth, meaning, vitality, and connectedness to others and the universe" (p. 128). Reed (1992) and Burkhardt (1994) expanded the theme of connectedness further and offered developmental views of spirituality that position the spiritual dimension of life squarely at the core of health and development across the lifespan.

## Spirituality and Health Care

Health care literature that addresses spirituality often reflects a tendency to medicalize this dimension of life. Heliker (1992) referred to spiritual distress as a "diagnostic category" in nursing (p. 16); as such, the term is used to label a patient's health problems and to guide nursing assessments and therapeutic planning. Patients are said to have "spiritual needs" and "spiritual problems" that must be diagnosed and treated appropriately (Highfield & Cason, 1983); treatment goals and interventions are discussed (Carson, 1989).

Within this medical framework, disagreement exists on how to approach the assessment of spirituality. In the nursing literature, Reed (1992) declared that "spirituality per se is not measurable any more than would be such concepts as *physicality, emotionality*, or *wholeness*" (p. 351). Carson (1989), however, stated that "Spiritual needs

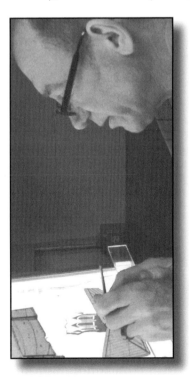

can be approached in the same systematic way that nurses approach biopsychosocial needs. The use of the nursing process, with its steps of assessment, analysis, planning, implementations, and evaluation, is quite applicable to spirituality" (p. 155). Highfield and Cason (1983) proposed a checklist of observable indicators of spiritual problems and spiritual health. Other assessment instruments in the literature include a Self-Test of Connectedness Possibilities (Bellingham et al., 1989), a Spiritual Well-Being Scale (Paloutzian & Ellison, 1982), and a variety of questionnaires, mapping strategies, and life scenario activities (Chapman, 1987; Hodge, 2005).

Again from nursing, Carson (1989) stated, "Probably the most effective spiritual intervention is the nurse's offering of self" (p. 163); to empathize, to listen, and to be available is to offer one's self to another. Benner (1984) spoke of this kind of intervention as "presencing" (p. 57); that is, being *fully present* to a client or patient by attentiveness, eye contact, touch, and silence. Presencing is an approach to care giving that may be especially relevant and important when caring for a dying person. Through presencing, the health care professional can help dissolve the feeling of separateness that so profoundly exists in the context of dying and death (Hasselkus, 1993).

A review of the previous literature from nursing and other journals of health promotion reveals the same tensions that exist within the literature on spirituality and occupational therapy—the struggle to define spirituality, the effort to include it under the umbrella of health and health care concerns, the ongoing discussion of its religious or nonreligious nature, the efforts by some and resistance by others to medicalize this phenomenon.

## SPIRITUALITY AND OCCUPATION: COMPATIBLE PARTNERS?

In 1991, the Canadian Association of Occupational Therapists published its model of occupational performance (CAOT, 1991); spirituality, defined as "the force that permeates and gives meaning to all life" (p. 142), was one of four performance components that comprised the model, along with the more familiar dimensions of self care, productivity, and leisure. At the time, the inclusion of spirituality in the Canadian model of occupational performance seemed a bold and somewhat startling step to many occupational therapists in other parts of the world, including my own country, the United States. As the Canadian document stated, "This component [spirituality] has rarely been identified in the previously cited American occupational therapy literature" (p. 18), but its early presence in the foundations of occupational therapy practice in Canada was declared.

Three years later, a special issue of the *Canadian Journal of Occupational Therapy (CJOT)* (1994, Vol. 61, No. 2) was devoted to the theme of "Spirituality and Occupation." Efforts were made in the special issue to conceptualize and define spirituality further so that its role in practice could be better operationalized (Egan & DeLaat, 1994; Urbanowski & Vargo, 1994). In the same year, the first volume of the *Journal of Occupational Science: Australia* was published. In an article in the third issue, do Rozario proposed that therapeutic activities that are anchored in the personal histories and rituals of people's lives foster rehabilitation; she likened the process of therapy to a spiritual journey, one that brings about spiritual reconciliation and transformation within the individual (do Rozario, 1994).

### A Wake-Up Call to Spirituality

In some ways, the emerging emphasis on spirituality evident in some of the occupational therapy literature, especially in Canada, served as a wake-up call to therapists in other parts of the world. A year after the publication of the 1994 special issue of *CJOT*, spirituality was included in a position paper on occupation approved by the American Occupational Therapy Association Representative Assembly (AOTA, 1995). In the AOTA paper, the spiritual nature of occupation was defined as the "nonphysical and nonmaterial aspects of existence" that contribute "insight into the nature and meaning of a person's life" (p. 1015). As can be seen, in attempting to gain access to

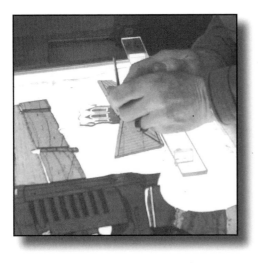

and define the spiritual nature of occupation, the authors of the position paper fell back on describing what it was *not*.

In 1997, a special issue of *The American Journal of Occupational Therapy (AJOT)* was published with the theme "Occupation, Spirituality, and Life Meaning" (Vol. 52, No. 6). In this issue, Christiansen referred to the "neglect of spirituality in U.S. occupational therapy" (p. 171) and called for acknowledgement of the spirituality of daily occupation and occupational therapy theory and practice.

Also in 1997, *The British Journal of Occupational Therapy (BJOT)* entered the dialogue by publishing a review of letters submitted over the previous 60 years (Kelly, 1997); highlighted was a series of letters spanning the years 1979 to 1996 that focused on spirituality and occupational therapy, largely within a religious context. The letters included a sometimes heated debate about whether or not spirituality relates only to formal religion, or could it be considered a human attribute outside the context of religion (and thus be a legitimate dimension of therapy). The letter exchange reflected personal definitions of spirituality in religious terms and included issues related to the "ethics" of incorporating Eastern philosophies such as yoga and zen into occupational therapy practice. One writer went so far as to refer to such practices as "heathen," to which other writers responded with "embarrassment," apologies to readers, and declarations that practices such as yoga represented not a religion but "a way of life" (Kelly, p. 437).

## More Controversy and Dissension

Meanwhile, the Canadian Association of Occupational Therapists further refined its emerging conceptualization of client-centered practice, proposing a new Canadian Model of Occupational Performance (CAOT, 1997). In the new model, "the importance of spirit (spirituality) in achieving the occupational potential of individuals and communities" is emphasized (Townsend, 1998). In reflecting on this model, Townsend stated, "[Canadian occupational therapists] are now locating spirituality as central to the person, shaped by the environment, and giving meaning to occupations" (p. 63). One dissenting *CJOT* reader (Smith, 1997) wrote a letter in reaction to the positioning of spirituality at the center of practice, stating, "I do not understand how one can possibly suggest that spirituality is at the centre of our profession ... it is more important to establish scientific research to support the existence of occupational therapy rather than a philosophical basis for the profession. I find it offensive that CAOT would allow its national publication to function as nothing more than a soapbox on which one can espouse personal beliefs" (p. 217). In stark contrast, Brockett (1997) commented in the same issue that the special spirituality issue of *CJOT* helped restore the "qualitative aspects of life or the 'art' of practice to its proper place" (p. 216). Brockett further stated, "I liken the process of occupational therapy to that of unlocking the potential for 'being' or becoming. ... We contribute to the process through 'doing,' using occupation to nurture and encourage the seed" (p. 216).

In 2002, and then again in 2005, the Australians joined the discussion, focusing on the relevance or irrelevance of spirituality to occupational therapy practice (Wilding, 2002; Wilding, May, & Muir-Cochrane, 2005). Finally, Canadian Hammell (2003) went further to suggest that the word spirituality be avoided altogether, proposing instead the term *intrinsicality* to stand for the concept of a personal philosophy of meaning in our daily lives. To Hammell, intrinsicality refers to "the notion of a personal philosophy of meaning that informs life choices and the meaning we give to and derive from our every-day lives" (p. 71).

The discomfort about spirituality in our professional practice is also evident in the findings from the national survey of occupational therapists in the United States conducted by Engquist, Short-DeGraff, Gliner, and Oltjenbruns (1997). In regard to therapists' beliefs and practices about spirituality and therapy, 89% of the respondents in their study felt that spirituality was an important part of their lives and 84% viewed spirituality as a very important dimension of health and rehabilitation, yet "less than 40% indicated that addressing clients' spiritual needs was within the scope of their professional practice" (p. 173). Reasons given by respondents for the gap between beliefs and practices were that "spirituality is so subjective" and the lack of "a definitive measure" of spirituality (p. 178). Very similar results were obtained in a British survey of occupational therapists published two years later (Rose, 1999). In a 2004 publication, Belcham added role ambiguity to the list of reasons for the gap, with a significant negative correlation found between "the clarity of role and the perceived difficulty in addressing religious/spiritual beliefs" (p. 43).

Thus, it can be seen that spirituality lies uneasily with occupation in our profession at this point in time, with views among therapists ranging all the way from wholesale exclusion of the concept from therapy to asserting that it is central to the meaning of occupation and therapeutic practice. Much of the debate stems from different views and definitions of spirituality, with one important issue being whether or not spirituality represents formal religion or a broader aspect of life. The foundational value of our profession centers on occupation; what, if anything, does an occupational view of the world have to offer to the realm of spirituality that is important and unique?

# SPIRITUALITY AND EVERYDAY OCCUPATION

In his 1996 book, *The Re-Enchantment of Everyday Life*, Thomas Moore defines enchantment as the potential catalyst for reuniting the interior and exterior aspects of life, for "the reconciliation of inner and outer" (p. 284). To Moore, enchantment is present in those moments of life "when the heart is overwhelmed by beauty and the imagination is electrified by some haunting quality in the world or by a spirit or voice speaking from deep within a thing, a place, or a person" (p. ix). Moore further stated that it is by giving concrete expression to this interior spirit or voice that we bring about this reconciliation, and that we are able to break down the barriers between the inside and the outside. So it is that creative expressions of art and poetry provide reconciliation of the spiritual with the external dimensions of our lives. One has only to think of the beautiful dot paintings of the Australian indigenous peoples to recognize a tangible expression of inner dreams and stories.

So, once again, we come upon the theme of "inner and outer" as a way to express the sense of two dimensions of life—the spiritual inner and the pragmatic outer. Moore (1996) moved the discussion closer to occupation and occupational therapy with his descriptions of how we can give expression to this interior voice and, in so doing, how we can reconcile the inner and outer dimensions of our lives. Although Moore is not an occupational therapist, he is, in essence, saying that it is through our creative expressions, that is, our creative *doing*, that we integrate and blend both dimensions of our lives.

To me, it is not a huge leap from this concept of creative doing as a concrete expression of spirituality in our lives to the corollary concept of *all* everyday occupation as the concrete expression of spirituality. Urbanowski and Vargo (1994) suggested this precisely when they defined spirituality as "the experience of meaning in everyday activities" (p. 91). In such a view, spirituality is embodied in the occupations of daily life, and it is through these everyday expressions of the self that the inner and outer dimensions of our lives can become one.

## Ordinary Occupation as Spiritual Expression

So now we have arrived at the connection between occupation and spirituality. In the view presented here, occupation is a vehicle—perhaps a *primary* vehicle—by which the interior and exterior dimensions of one's self are reconciled, are integrated, are united, and expressed as a whole. Yerxa (1998) referred to this phenomenon as "the human spirit for occupation" (p. 412). Peloquin raised this point in her editorial introduction to the spirituality issue of *The American Journal of Occupational Therapy* (Peloquin, 1997). Occupation is a form of *making*, and it is this dimension of occupation that expresses the spiritual self. To illustrate her meaning, Peloquin quoted a poem, the last two lines of which were:

> So much of who I am
> is subtly spoken in my making. (Petersen, 1976)

That is to say, what I make, create, bring into being, is an expression of my own being—is "so much of who I am." The spirit of the inner room emerges via ordinary but creative occupations such as knitting, making a meal, writing a letter, learning a new computer program, holding a conversation. Occupations bring about connections with the self, others, the environment, or, for some, a sense of a higher Being. This is compatible with Peloquin's (1997) view, that occupation is an act of making, and this act of making "is one in which human *being* (character, heart, spirit) flows into human *doing*" (p. 168, emphasis added). Meaningful occupation may thus be seen as a phenomenon that "animates and extends the human spirit" (p. 167).

In my research on occupation and well-being in people with dementia (Hasselkus, 1998), one of the daycare staff respondents in the study described the experience of a participant in a cooking group in a way that revealed the woman's fragile, but still vital, spirituality:

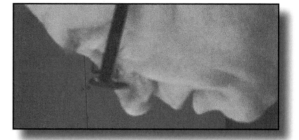

> She could not get the supplies ready herself, but if we would have the supplies sitting out for her—like the half a cup of butter, and the two cups of flour, and the brown sugar—she could mix that up. I mean, she just—she *glowed*. And she would talk about it and then she would reminisce about her cooking days. And she could take teaspoons of the cookie dough and drop them on the cookie sheet and just talk. And she would just smile. She would just become *radiant*. (p. 429)

One might say that, in this story, the occupation of making cookies animated and extended the spirit of the participant; the woman "glowed" and became "radiant" and reminisced about her cooking days. The occupation of cooking was one in which this person's inner being emerged and flowed into her doing. The cooking was the catalyst that opened the door, enabling the spirit of her inner room to burst forth into the outer world. To paraphrase Susan Lydon's (1997) comment about her knitting passion, for the woman with dementia, the important thing was not so much what she cooked but what happened to her while she cooked it.

Putting it another way, Moore (1996) stated, "We are made up not of many parts, as though we were mechanical objects, but rather of an infinite number of stories" (p. 201). We can think of those stories as residing deep within us, part of our inner spiritual beings. Occupation helps in the continual creation of new stories and it helps to give us access to existing stories. Using this metaphor, we might say that the daycare participant held within herself rich stories of cooking, created from her household activities earlier in life. Cooking in the group at the daycare center provided access to stories deep within her, facilitating the release of those stories for re-living in the present.

In Jacques and Hasselkus' (2004) study of the meaning of occupation surrounding dying and death, one of the conclusions drawn from the 6-month study in a residential hospice was that the nature of familiar and even ordinary occupations seemed charged with enlarged meanings in the presence of dying and impending death. For example, Mark, one of the residents of the hospice, was visited by his granddaughter and her husband one evening; Jacques wrote in her journal, "They shared his favorite pie and watched a favorite game show on television while they played cards. Their easy manner and laughter suggested this had been a familiar routine for them before Mark's admission to the hospice residence" (p. 48). This domestic scene can be interpreted as an example of Mark being able to live out one of his inner stories, while dying. When another resident, Daniel, was very close to death, his girlfriend mentioned that he always "liked to cuddle," so the nurse and aide made room for her to be next to him on the bed (p. 50); she stayed at the hospice with him until he died 3 days later. Ordinary occupations such as these are infused with a special poignancy and meaning in the context of dying; "Occupations at the end of life are framed within the experience of dying" (p. 51).

## Gaining Intimacy With Our Inner Stories

We all use occupation in many different ways to gain intimacy with our inner stories—our spirituality. Mary Forhan's (2010) beautifully written autoethnography of her lived experience of grief and loss when her full-term son was stillborn offers a moving narrative of the meaning of everyday occupation in such a heart-wrenching journey. As she searched to understand the story she was living, Forhan engaged in writing a journal describing her personal experience and occupational responses to the emotional pain and deep grief of the situation. In other words, she sought to put her inner story into words and then to convey that story to a wider audience of occupational therapists through her journal article.

Somewhat similarly, Hoppes and Segal (2010) studied occupational responses to mourning and bereavement after a family member's death. Occupational strategies used by participants in their study after the death included accommodations in work and leisure ("After she passed away … I left the job I'd been at for 13 years. I thought, 'You know, I don't need this.' You just look at the world differently"; p. 236); increased importance of familiar friendships and routines ("Doing things with our friends has always been a priority. We derive a lot of strength from that. Our friends now are closer to us"; p. 238); and maintenance of bonds with the deceased family member through occupations such as care of the deceased's possessions or continued involvement in an occupation valued by the person who has died ("I played softball all through college … and the grandfather I was very close to came to all my games. So that was really important after he passed away that I continue to do that. It almost had more importance afterwards" (p. 239).

In the guest bedroom of my home, I have a small antique chest of drawers in which I have arranged a collection of my grandmother's sewing items. In the top drawer, I have placed her wooden crochet hooks, knitting needles, darning egg, and tatting shuttle with a piece of lace tatting still attached—all items she brought from Sweden when she and my grandfather emigrated to the United States in 1894. In another drawer, I keep her handmade wooden hairpin lace frames and samples of hairpin lace. In the third drawer, I have her pincushions, scissors, and thimbles.

The sewing items of my grandmother represent one of my inner stories; I "visit" them regularly—touching each one, rearranging them; they contribute in a gentle way to my continued search for myself in this life. There is a spirit in the items, present for me, but probably not present, at least not in the same way, for anyone else on earth. Sexson (1992) might refer to my collection of items as a "sacred text" (p. 29); that is, it serves as a means of understanding my inner self and my relationship to the world of meaning. Each time I look over my collection and handle the lovely things brought all the way from Sweden more than a century ago, the women of my family are there with me—my grandmother, my mother, my sister. I understand a little better who they were. I understand a little better who I am. I "belong," and I continue to "become."

In her article on heirlooms as special objects, Irene Ilott (2006) stated that these objects have multiple meanings in our lives, reflecting personal, societal, and cultural levels; "Heirlooms are tangible evidence of both existence and continuity across generations" (p. 145). Family heirlooms serve as "tangible evidence of domestic history"; they are representations of past achievements and skills, objects "embedded in a specific social network" (p. 148). And, as Ilott said, family members are guardians rather than owners of such objects. All of this holds true for me and the keepsakes from my Swedish grandmother—they are tangible evidence of my family's domestic history, they represent past achievements and skills, and they are embedded in the social network of my family. They are stories that lie deep within me.

# SPIRITUALITY AND OCCUPATIONAL THERAPY

Moore (1996) stated that, spirituality is like "a lowly emanation from the most humble and earthbound things" (p. 339). There is, of course, also a spirituality that aims higher, finding its expression in the towering steeples of temples and churches and in lofty mountain peaks. But it seems likely that it is in the earthbound things—the pincushions and thimbles of our everyday lives—that spirituality finds its connection with occupational *therapy*. The spirituality of occupational therapy emanates from the therapeutic experiences embodied in everyday occupations.

## Occupation as a Release of Spirit

In occupational therapy, we focus on enabling clients to engage in occupation. We believe that this engagement in occupation relates in a positive way to each client's health and well-being. Above, I have presented one view of occupation as a vehicle for, in effect, *releasing* or *freeing* a person's spiritual being. From this view, engagement in occupation serves as an agent that activates and provides expression for a person's spiritual self in the world. If the ability to experience the spirituality of one's life is an aspect of one's health and well-being (and there are those who would say it is the essence of health and well-being), then occupational therapy provides a vehicular context "from which spiritual experiences or well-being may occur" (Collins, 1998, p. 281).

Ramugondo (2005) spoke of "unlocking spirituality" through the use of play in her study of mothering a child with HIV/AIDS in Cape Town, South Africa. In her project, she led workshops in which participants (mothers) explored ways to promote "play, playfulness, and caregiver involvement in the interaction between the caregiver and the child" (p. 316). In the study, the mothers gained understandings about the healthful benefits of play for both themselves and their children, many having started the project with beliefs that a sick child should not play, that play required purchased toys, and that they themselves did not have a role as enablers of play. That play facilitated the release of spirit in the mothers and children is illustrated in a quote from one of the participant mothers: "Yes I get it! When my child plays, she's happy, and when she is happy, she looks healthy, and I am happy" (p. 318).

Egan and DeLaat (1994) expressed this view very clearly in their article on spirituality in occupational therapy practice: "The spirit is seen as the essence of the person. In

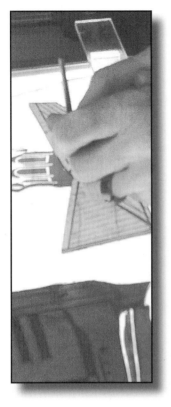

this way the spirit cannot be made more healthy, it can only be allowed more freedom through a strengthening or adjustment to the tools which it uses to express itself" (p. 101). This statement touches directly on a source of tension in the continuing discussions about spirituality and occupational therapy. As an example of a different view, Rosenfeld, at the turn of this century, made efforts to "fit" spirituality into the existing structure of occupational therapy, referring to spirituality as a "modality" and using concepts of occupational performance areas, components and context to define it (2000, 2001). Tension exists between those health professionals who accept spirituality as a legitimate part of practice that can be molded into the traditional medical framework and those who view spirituality not as another aspect of a person that may be unhealthy and in need of treatment but rather as an aspect of a person that can be encouraged and helped to express itself by certain therapeutic experiences.

This tension was evident to me at the 1998 World Federation of Occupational Therapists' 12th Congress in Montreal. I was present at a roundtable discussion on spirituality. With this audience of therapists from all around the world, discussion ranged across how to teach spirituality, how to assist students to find their own spirituality, how to use rituals and journaling in therapy to enhance spirituality, how to define spirituality as occupation, and, yes, how to assess spirituality. Perhaps in exasperation, one member of the audience finally stood up and expressed his own Eastern view of the spirit. He stated strongly that spirituality is not something to separate out from other parts of life, to assess, or to try to "improve"; rather, spirituality is a life process to be recognized and lived. We may, through our occupational therapy, enhance a person's ability to "live" their spirituality; but, in this man's view, spirituality is not something we can isolate, measure, or seek to improve. Nor should we even try.

Collins (1998) reflected a similar view when he referred to occupation as an "antecedent" for spiritual experiences (p. 281). To Collins, the quality of the experience in occupational therapy serves as a wellspring from which spiritual experiences and well-being may arise. He offered his own suggestions for ways to develop the quality of the experience that occurs in therapy, emphasizing the importance of a therapist developing a deep awareness of the contextual experiences of a client's life. Understanding clients' values, feelings about themselves and what they do, the forms that their occupations take, and their occupational plans for the future "may help to create awareness of spiritual expression in daily life activities or experiences" (p. 182).

Alternatively, while Brockelman (2002) offered a similar view of the potential for occupation to be a freeing agent for spiritual expression, he also proposed some exceptions—namely, that deeply ingrained everyday habits and routines can, in fact, act as *barriers* to spiritual renewal and personal growth. To Brockelman, habitual attitudes and behaviors can be constricting and inadequate; spiritual growth can occur only through a "letting go" of these habits and attitudes, an act that "opens a person to new and liberating ways of living and being in the world" (p. 29S). A therapist might work with a client to facilitate this "letting go," thus enabling the client to experience a sense of liberation and possibility in his or her life. Wallenbert and Jonsson (2005) addressed the "pull" of prior habits against adaptation and change in their research on clients' experiences in rehabilitation following stroke—citing the participants preferences for "waiting to get better, waiting for another solution, and waiting for the treatment to make an impact" (p. 218). Though not specifically addressing spiritual renewal, this research takes an innovative look at habits as they constrain openness to new ways of being in the world. Experiences in therapy that incorporate these contextual understandings may strengthen a client's ability to "live" his or her spiritual life.

Tensions continue to exist between those who conceptualize spirituality in treatment terms and those who understand spirituality more as a life force that does not lend itself to our occupational definitions or to our health care concepts. As recently as 2006, Thompson and MacNeil reported findings from a study of occupational therapy students in a seminar on spirituality; the students' concerns about spirituality related to a perceived "underlying clash between social and medical models of disability" were a prominent part of the findings. The conversation continues.

## The Narrative Structure of Spirituality

One final point related to this discussion of spirituality and occupational therapy has to do with the meaning of narrative within the profession. In earlier chapters, I have described the concept of narrative as it relates to meaning-making and therapist-client relationships. Narrative is the structure we give to life experiences as we live them, reflect on them, and relate them to others (Bruner, 1990; Polkinghorne, 1988). Narrative and its potential power to enhance the therapeutic experience in occupational therapy has been described and researched by others (Clark, 1993; Helfrich & Kielhofner, 1994; Mattingly, 1998). Kirsh and Welch (2003) further extended narrative theory and describe the power of narrative in therapy situations to reveal a client's spirituality. According to Kirsh and Welch, creating a narrative requires framing and reframing, selection and ordering of one's life; these cognitive activities can lead to enriched thinking about life's purpose and meaning. Thus, the use of narrative in therapy may actually enhance a client's ability to express his or her spiritual essence.

A 2001 newspaper story (Brixey) illustrates this concept of narrative and spirituality very well. The long-time dean of one of the University of Wisconsin system's two-year campuses—a well-liked and effective administrator—announced, unexpectedly, his plans to retire. In describing his plans, the dean said that his decision came to him when he was recently visiting his daughter and her family in New Mexico. He is quoted as saying, "I was holding my grandson in my arms and watching the angle of the light. I felt like that little boy kind of whispered mortality to me and I knew there were some things yet I wanted to do." I was struck by the spiritual nature of this man's experience and by his ability to express it in narrative. Clearly, the moment in New Mexico while holding his grandson was a moment of reframing and reordering in his life. This man's spirituality seems clearly revealed in the brief story. The spiritual moment occurred in and, one could say, was *released by* the occupational context of grandfather and grandson being together during a family visit.

It seems a small step from thinking about the power of narrative to help understand a client's spirituality to interpreting the power of narrative within the context used earlier in the chapter— the metaphor of the inside room and the outside room. If narrative is a phenomenon that reveals meanings about one's life, then it is a phenomenon that reveals a person's "inside room." It is, in the context of the metaphor, one way to open the door between the inside and outside rooms and to thereby come to understand the meaning of the inside room and, thus, the person's spirituality.

## The Therapist's Own Spirit

Up to this point in the discussion of spirituality and occupational therapy, I have focused on the therapeutic process and the spirituality of the client. But as Thibeault (1996) has reminded us, the therapeutic process includes the therapeutic alliance of client *and* therapist. The importance of the therapist's own spirituality and well-being in the therapeutic transaction has been recognized by some (Collins, 1998; Egan & DeLaat, 1994, 1997; Egan & Swedersky, 2003; Hasselkus & Dickie, 1994; Kirsh, 1996; Rosa & Hasselkus, 1996, 2005).

In their earlier work, Egan and DeLaat (1994) advised therapists to "pay attention to your own spirit and nurture its expression" (p. 101). The therapeutic process comprises a transactional situation, experienced by both therapist and client. Of course, the process is also experienced by family, friends, and other professionals. Transactions need to be open to discovery of meanings and understandings (Kirsh, 1996). Beliefs about health and occupation apply to therapist as well as to client; "… both parties grow through the client-therapist relationship (Egan & DeLaat, 1997, p. 120). Once stated, this recognition of the therapist's needs and quality of experience in the therapeutic process seems self-evident. In the study by my graduate student (Jacques & Hasselkus, 2004), some of the staff at the residential hospice said that their everyday work had spiritual qualities, with one staff member stating that her work felt "like a ministry … a sacred time" (p. 51). The therapist's spiritual health or spiritual distress has implications for the growth and well-being of the therapist's self as well as implications for job satisfaction, career decisions, and retention and attrition in the profession. Yet the well-being of occupational therapists remains a relatively unexplored phenomenon. Further research on the relationship between spirituality and occupation will contribute to our understanding of not only our clients, but also of our selves.

## THE SPACE WITHIN

In his essay on spirituality and knowing, Huebner (1985) stated, "Every mode of knowing is a mode of being open, vulnerable, and available to the *internal* and *external* world … There is always a better way of being in the world, more complete prediction, more perfect expression of experience and feeling, more just meetings with others, better techniques and instrumentalities" (p. 170, emphasis added). Engagement in occupation is one primary way for us to "be" in the world. We can think of occupation as a vehicle by which our spiritual consciousness is given expression in our daily worldly lives.

In Lynne Sharon Schwartz's (1995) novel *The Fatigue Artist*, the tai chi teacher offers this: "Chinese art did make beautiful things, poems, paintings, pottery, all of them with a great deal of empty space. The empty space represents the inner life, what is most important but unseen. Like the breath, which is invisible but sustains us. … The space in a bowl, for instance. … You use the clay to make it, and that is the part you see, but what makes the bowl useful is the space within" (p. 126).

For our purposes, perhaps we can modify the last phrase of the tai chi master's saying to be, "What makes *life meaningful* is the space within." As occupational therapists, our use of occupation both gives us *access* to the space within and enables the *expression* of the vitality within that inner space. Remember the daycare participant with dementia and the cooking activity: "… she could take teaspoons of the cookie dough and drop them on the cookie sheet and just talk. And she would just smile. She would just become *radiant*."

# REFERENCES

American Occupational Therapy Association. (1995). Position paper: Occupation. *American Journal of Occupational Therapy, 49,* 1015-1018.

Banks, R. (1980). Health and the spiritual dimension: Relationships and implications for professional preparation programs. *Journal of School Health, 50,* 195-202.

Belcham, C. (2004). Spirituality in occupational therapy: Theory in practice? *British Journal of Occupational Therapy, 67,* 39-46.

Bellingham, R., Cohen, B., Jones, T., & Spaniol, L. (1989). Connectedness: Some skills for spiritual health. *American Journal of Health Promotion, 4,* 18-24.

Benner, P. (1984). *From novice to expert*. Menlo Park, CA: Addison-Wesley.

Brixey, E. (2001). UW-Richland's likable Kempthorne retiring. *Wisconsin State Journal,* p. 1.

Brockett, M. (1997). Spirituality issue affirms and challenges our thinking. *Canadian Journal of Occupational Therapy, 64,* 216.

Brockelman, P. T., (2002). Habits and personal growth: The art of the possible. *OTJR: Occupation, Participation and Health, 22*(Suppl. 1), 18S-30S.

Bruner, J. (1990). *Acts of meaning*. Cambridge, MA: Harvard University Press.

Burkhardt, M. A. (1994). Becoming and connecting: Elements of spirituality for women. *Holistic Nursing Practice, 8*(4), 12-21.

Canadian Association of Occupational Therapists. (1991). *Occupational therapy guidelines for client-centred practice*. Toronto, Ontario, Canada: CAOT Publishers.

Canadian Association of Occupational Therapy. (1997). *Enabling occupation: An occupational therapy perspective*. Ottawa, Ontario, Canada: CAOT Publishers, ACE.

Carson, V. B. (1989). Spirituality and the nursing process. In V. B. Carson (Ed.), *Spiritual dimensions of nursing practice* (pp. 150-179). Philadelphia, PA: W. B. Saunders.

Chapman, L. S. (1986). Spiritual health: A component missing from health promotion. *American Journal of Health Promotion, 1,* 38-41.

Chapman, L. S. (1987). Developing a useful perspective on spiritual health: Well-being, spiritual potential and the search for meaning. *American Journal of Health Promotion, 2,* 31-39.

Christiansen, C. (1997). Acknowledging a spiritual dimension in occupational therapy practice. *American Journal of Occupational Therapy, 51,* 169-172.

Clark F. (1993). Occupation imbedded in real life: Interweaving occupational science and occupational therapy. *American Journal of Occupational Therapy, 47,* 1067-1078.

Collins, M. (1998). Occupational therapy and spirituality: Reflecting on quality of experience in therapeutic interventions. *British Journal of Occupational Therapy, 61,* 280-284.

do Rosario, L. (1994). Ritual, meaning and transcendence: The role of occupation in modern life. *Journal of Occupational Science: Australia, 1*(3), 46-53.

Egan, M., & DeLaat, M. D. (1994). Considering spirituality in occupational therapy practice. *Canadian Journal of Occupational Therapy, 61,* 95-101.

Egan, M., & DeLaat, M. D. (1997). The implicit spirituality of occupational therapy practice. *Canadian Journal of Occupational Therapy, 64,* 115-121.

Egan, M., & Swedersky, J. (2003). Spirituality as experienced by occupational therapists in practice. *American Journal of Occupational Therapy, 57,* 525-533.

Engquist, D. E., Short-DeGraff, M., Gliner, J., & Oltjenbruns, K. (1997). Occupational therapists' beliefs and practices with regard to spirituality and therapy. *American Journal of Occupational Therapy, 51,* 173-180.

Forhan, M. (2010). Doing, being and becoming: A family's journey through perinatal loss. *American Journal of Occupational Therapy, 64,* 142-151.

Fowler, J. W. (1981). *Stages of faith: The psychology of human development and the quest for meaning.* San Francisco, CA: Harper & Row.

Hammell, K. W. (2003). Intrinsicality: Reflections on meanings and mandates. In M. A. McColl (Ed.), *Spirituality and occupational therapy* (pp. 67-82). Ottawa, Ontario: CAOT Publications ACE.

Hasselkus, B. R. (1993). Death in very old age: A personal journey of caregiving. *American Journal of Occupational Therapy, 47,* 717-723.

Hasselkus, B. R. (1998). Occupation and well-being in dementia: The experience of day-care staff. *American Journal of Occupational Therapy, 52,* 423-434.

Hasselkus, B. R., & Dickie, V. A. (1994). Doing occupational therapy: Dimensions of satisfaction and dissatisfaction. *American Journal of Occupational Therapy, 48,* 145-154.

Helfrich, C., & Kielhofner, G. (1994). Volitional narratives and the meaning of therapy. *American Journal of Occupational Therapy, 48,* 319-326.

Heliker, D. (1992). Reevaluation of a nursing diagnosis: Spiritual distress. *Nursing Forum, 27*(4), 15-20.

Highfield, M. F., & Cason, C. (1983). Spiritual needs of patients: Are they recognized. *Cancer Nursing, 6,* 187-192.

Hodge, D. R. (2005). Spiritual lifemaps: A client-centered pictorial instrument for spiritual assessment, planning, and intervention. *Social Work, 50,* 77-87.

Hoppes, S., & Segal, R. (2010). Reconstructing meaning through occupation after the death of a family member: Accommodation, assimilation, and continuing bonds. *American Journal of Occupational Therapy, 64,* 133-141.

Huebner, D. E. (1985). Spirituality and knowing. In E. Eisner (Ed.), *Learning and teaching the ways of knowing* (pp. 159-173). Chicago, IL: University of Chicago Press.

Ilott, I. (2006). A special occupation: Commissioning an heirloom. *Journal of Occupational Science, 13,* 145-148.

Jacques, N., & Hasselkus, B. R. (2004). The nature of occupation surrounding dying and death. *OTJR: Occupation, Participation and Health, 24,* 44-53.

Kelly, G. (1997). Letters to the editor: The last 60 years. *British Journal of Occupational Therapy, 60,* 436-440.

Kirsh, B. (1996). A narrative approach to addressing spirituality in occupational therapy: Exploring personal meaning and purpose. *Canadian Journal of Occupational Therapy, 63,* 55-61.

Kirsh, B., & Welch, A. (2003). Opening the door to spiritual expression: The power of narrative in occupational therapy. In M. A. McColl (Ed.), *Spirituality and occupational therapy* (pp. 161-180). Ottawa, Ontario, Canada: CAOTA Publications, ACE.

Lydon, S. G. (1997). *The knitting sutra: Craft as a spiritual practice.* San Francisco, CA: Harper Collins.

Mattingly, C. (1998). *Healing dramas and clinical plots: The narrative structure of experience.* Cambridge, UK: Cambridge University Press.

McColl, M. A. (Ed.). (2003). *Spirituality and occupational therapy.* Ottawa, Ontario: CAOT Publications, ACE.

McCullers, C. (1940). *The heart is a lonely hunter.* New York, NY: Houghton Mifflin.

McFadden, S. H., & Gerl, R. R (1990). Approaches to understanding spirituality in the second half of life. *Generations,* 35-38.

Miller, J. F. (1985). Assessment of loneliness and spiritual well-being in chronically ill and healthy adults. *Journal of Professional Nursing, 1,* 79-85.

Moore, T. (1996). *The re-enchantment of everyday life.* New York, NY: Harper Collins.

Morphy, H. (1998). *Aboriginal art.* London, UK: Phaidon Press United.

Paloutzian, R., & Ellison, C. (1982). Loneliness, spiritual well-being, and quality of life. In L. Peplau & D. Perlman (Eds.), *Loneliness: A sourcebook of current theory, research, and therapy* (pp. 224-237). New York, NY: John Wiley & Sons.

Peloquin, S. M. (1997). The spiritual depth of occupation: Making worlds and making lives. *American Journal of Occupational Therapy, 51,* 167-168.

Petersen, J. (1976). *The book of yes.* Niles, IL: Argus.

Polkinghorne, D. E. (1988). *Narrative knowing and the human sciences.* Albany, NY: SUNY Press.

Pollner, M. (1989). Divine relations, social relations, and well-being. *Journal of Health & Social Behavior, 30,* 92-104.

Ramugondo, E. L. (2005). Unlocking spirituality: Play as a health-promoting occupation in the context of HIV/AIDS. In F. Kronenberg, S. S. Algado, & N. Pollard, (Eds.), *Occupational therapy without borders: Learning from the spirit of survivors* (pp. 313-325). New York, NY: Elsevier.

Reed, P. G. (1992). An emerging paradigm for the investigation of spirituality in nursing. *Research in Nursing Health, 15,* 349-357.

Rosa, S., & Hasselkus, B. R. (1996). Connecting with patients: The personal experience of professional helping. *Occupational Therapy Journal of Research, 16,* 245-260.

Rosa, S., & Hasselkus, B. R. (2005). Finding common ground with patients: The centrality of compatibility. *American Journal of Occupational Therapy, 59,* 198-208.

Rose, A. (1999). Spirituality and palliative care: The attitudes of occupational therapists. *British Journal of Occupational Therapists, 62,* 307-312.

Rosenfeld, M. S. (2000). Spiritual agent modalities for occupational therapy practice. *OT Practice,* 17-21.

Rosenfeld, M. S. (2001). Exploring a spiritual context for care. *OT Practice,* 18-25.

Schwartz, L. S. (1995). *The fatigue artist.* New York, NY: Scribner.

Sexson, L. (1992). *Ordinarily sacred.* Charlottesville, VA: University Press of Virginia.

Smith, L. (1997). Letter to the editor: Spirituality questioned as profession's centre. *Canadian Journal of Occupational Therapy, 64,* 217.

Stiles, M. K. (1990). The shining stranger: Nurse-family spiritual relationships. *Cancer Nursing, 13,* 235-245.

Stoll, R. I. (1989). The essence of spirituality. In V. B. Carson (Ed.), *Spiritual dimensions of nursing practice* (pp. 4-23). Philadelphia, PA: W. B. Saunders.

Sullivan, W. P. (1993). "It helps me to be a whole person": The role of spirituality among the mentally challenged. *Psychosocial Rehabilitation Journal, 16,* 125-134.

Thibeault, R. (1996). *The client-centred guidelines: Help! I have lost myself and my spirit is gone!* Paper presented at the Canadian Association of Occupational Therapists Annual Conference.

Thompson, B. E., & MacNeil, C. (2006). A phenomenological study exploring the meaning of a seminar on spirituality for occupational therapy students. *American Journal of Occupational Therapy, 60,* 531-539.

Townsend, E. (1998). Client-centred occupational therapy: The Canadian experience. In M. Law (Ed.), *Client-centered occupational therapy* (pp. 47-64). Thorofare, NJ: SLACK Incorporated.

Urbanowski, R., & Vargo, J. (1994). Spirituality, daily practice, and the occupational performance model. *Canadian Journal of Occupational Therapy, 61,* 88-94.

Wallenbert, I., & Jonsson, H. (2005). Waiting to get better: A dilemma regarding habits in daily occupations after stroke. *American Journal of Occupational Therapy, 59,* 218-224.

Wilding, C. (2002). Where angels fear to tread: Is spirituality relevant to occupational therapy practice? *Australian Occupational Therapy Journal, 49,* 44-47.

Wilding, C., May, E., & Muir-Cochrane, E. (2005). Experience of spirituality, mental illness and occupation: A life-sustaining phenomenon. *Australian Occupational Therapy Journal, 52,* 1-9.

Yerxa, E. (1998). Health and the human spirit for occupation. *American Journal of Occupational Therapy, 52,* 412-418.

# CHAPTER 9

# CREATIVITY IN OCCUPATION AS A SOURCE OF MEANING

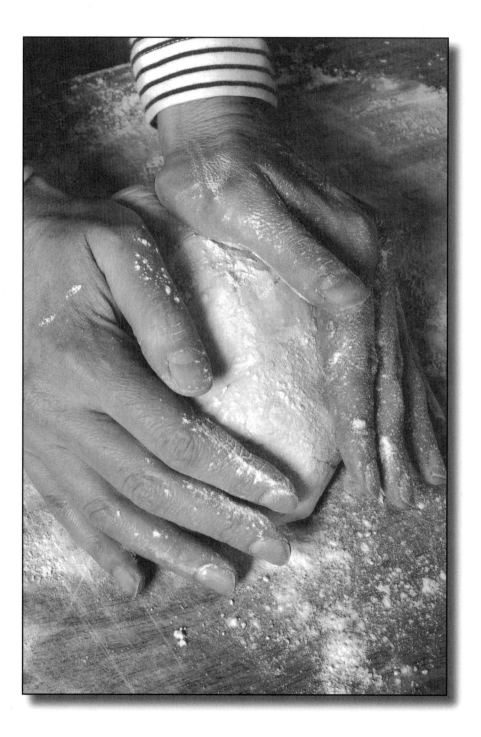

When we speak of creativity, of what exactly do we speak?

Runco and Richards (1997, p. ix)

Creative moments and acts are often recognizable in our lives, yet in our attempts to explain and understand what creativity is, we fall back on metaphors, such as saying a person is "able to think outside the box," or is "marching to a different drummer," or that something is "a horse of a different color." James, Clark, and Cropanzano (1999) defined *creativity* as the "generation and elaboration of ideas or products" that are novel, useful, and goal directed (p. 211). Being "novel" means representing some type of departure from what existed or was known previously; according to James et al., novelty is the crucial element of creativity.

Wilcock (2006) described creativity as "one of the most complex of human capacities" (p. 120). She cited particular traits used to characterize creative people such as intuition, spontaneity, flexibility, openness, and independence. Myers, in her book on the creative process, said that, "Creativity is an intimidating word. Strong. Powerful" (1999, p. xiii). I agree. Yet, Myers also said that creativity can be said to be "something of everyday life" (p. xiii).

It is the creativity of everyday life that I want to explore in this chapter, what Cohen (2000) referred to as "creativity with a little c" (p. 263). At the heart of creativity with a "little c" is the ability to "recognize in the complexity of life the infinite opportunities for new ideas and interactions, and the power of small changes to bring about larger ones" (p. 263). Everyday creativity represents a departure from the view of creativity as represented only in exceptional and rare accomplishment such as was found in great artists or great performers. As Dickie said, "… the elevation of creativity to the status of something only a few might attain constrains others from engaging in creative occupations" (2004, p. 56). Everyday creativity also moves beyond traditional creative realms such as the arts and the humanities. In everyday creativity, creativity is considered a quality or capability that is present to varying degrees in all human beings and that potentially manifests itself in virtually all aspects of daily life (Blanche, 2007; Dickie; Goff, 1997; McNiff, 1998; Richards, Kinney, Lunde, Benet, & Merzel, 1997; SARK, 1999).

Runco and Richards (1997) said, "We do not for a minute intend to minimize the importance of eminent and exceptional accomplishments, particularly in the arts and sciences, which many people identify first with 'creativity.' … Yet we look beyond these as well, to creativity as a general style of thinking, even of living. Of the essence of *originality* brought to the tasks of everyday life. Of creativity as an essential tool for adaptation to our environment and, indeed, to a changing world. Creativity, when viewed this way, becomes an essential survival tool, and not just for a few people, but for everyone" (p. ix).

Occupation, too, is a phenomenon that pervades daily life. To writers such as Peloquin (1997), much of daily occupation is composed of creating—acts of making; "The objects of human making, not just the tangibles like belts or splints, but the less tangible like friendship and discovery, extend the world and show the human share in creation" (p. 167). For Peloquin, it is through everyday occupation that the power of creation and creativity are revealed.

Hasselkus, B. R.
*The Meaning of Everyday Occupation, Second Edition* (pp. 165-182).
© 2011 SLACK Incorporated

# CREATIVITY FROM WITHOUT AND WITHIN

So where *does* it come from—this creativity? In this chapter, I will explore these and other ideas about the origins and the experience of creativity in our lives and the relationship of everyday creativity to health and occupation. What is the primordial source for the genesis of originality and novelty in our lives? From her philosophical perspective, Myers (1999) declared that *inspiration* is the starting point of all creative acts; "Inspiration breathes the creative soul into our minds and our hearts" (p. xv). But what is inspiration? And what is the source of inspiration?

## Starting With Our Surroundings

When I first set out to write this book, I was already in the throes of creating a writing "place"—a place that would support and encourage my thinking and, yes, my creativity. Since moving into our house 10 years earlier, I had been somewhat less than thrilled about the basement location for my "office" and the hodgepodge of office-type leftover furniture that comprised the trappings. Ultimately, my desire to upgrade the ambiance of the space led first to the acquisition of new office furnishings with built-in files, desktops, drawers, and lots of good flat surface space to spread out my books, papers, and journals. At the same time, we had new lighting installed in the ceiling above the work surfaces. Next came a new computer with a speaker system and a CD drive; for the first time in my life, I could conveniently play music while I wrote. Next came a new built-in bookshelf to supplement my desk space and to house my growing stacks of materials now being organized by chapters. Lastly, I decided at some point, somewhat self-consciously, that I would like to have a candle burning while I wrote, and so the final and most modest touch was the purchase of a supply of candles—big, thick ones that smell like vanilla and that burn a long time. Now when I am ready for a few hours of writing, I sort of settle in, put on the music of my choice, light my candle, and hope for a productive, inspired session in the special space I have created.

In some ways, perhaps one's physical environment acts like a birth mother, providing the host entity and sustenance that enable creativity to be born and to flourish. Feldhusen and Goh (1995) stated that for each individual, "there is an optimum fit with the environment" (p. 233) that supports the essence of creativity. Of course, the flip side of such a statement is that many environments will *not* be optimum supports for creativity. Toomey said, "Creativity is particularly sensitive to those components that surround the activity. … When both the creative and the spiritual aspects of the person, place, and task are in harmony, then the endeavor can take on a life of its own, the work will occur in the moment, and original and new things will happen" (2003, p. 190). I have worked on my space for writing to bring about a place for myself that feels like a good fit, the best I can do. What constitutes an "optimum fit" will obviously vary from individual to individual.

SARK (1999) has said, "We need some space to make our creative dreams real" (p. 42). Yet, little is known about just how a space enables us to realize our creative dreams. What are the interrelationships and interdependencies between one's surroundings and one's creativity? What is it about my basement space that now feels like it supports my creative endeavors, but that was missing prior to all the changes? My guess is that the writing space is, first of all, a space that is truly mine—it is a "room" of my own. No one else uses it. I have not had to actually declare this to anyone; apparently, the space speaks for itself. Secondly, I suppose that, because we live in a materialistic society, the new sleek furnishings send me and those around me the message that what I am doing in this space is important and to be respected, that my writing is an occupation that is deserving of the time and energy and resources devoted to the planning and changes in the make-up of this space. Thirdly, as SARK also said, "Creativity adores solitude" (p. 41). In accord with these words, my most creative work seems to be done when I am in this space alone—in solitude. In my best solitary moments, I like to think that I can hear what Cassou (1999) called "the heartbeat of creativity" (p. 2). I become "lost" in the writing, unaware of the passage of time and oblivious to things beyond my immediate space. When the nearby telephone suddenly rings, I lurch in my chair, reluctantly tear my eyes away from the words, words, words in which I have been so absorbed, and return to the world. The creative moment, "filled with spirit" (Cassou, p. 5), is no more. But that is all right; as Cassou also said, creativity breathes in and out, as does the rest of life, and there will be more moments filled with spirit in the days ahead.

The nature of the physical environment that surrounds us seems to be one of the determinants of creativity. It remains something of a mystery as to just how the characteristics of the environment interact with the individual to generate creative behavior (Harrington, 1990; Mace, 1997); yet, I know that the specially planned space that I now have for writing somehow contributes to my productivity and creativity during the time I spend there.

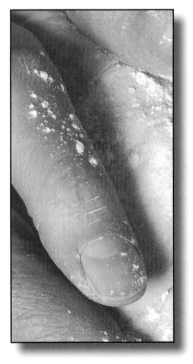

## Creativity and the Social World

Creativity is regarded by some as not so much an expression of solitude as a phenomenon within a social world. Dickie (2004), in her engaging article on creativity and quilting, spoke of the *community* of quilters as a major source of support for creativity; "Quilters tend to clump together. They join guilds, critique groups … they sew alongside each other, learning together at workshops, sharing ideas and teaching one another …" (p. 56). Dickie rightly pointed out that even those quilters who work alone are connected to social networks as they select fabric, give away or sell completed quilts, exhibit quilts, etc. The emphasis by some in this relational view of creativity is on the influence of the opportunities and constraints of the *social* milieu on the creative process (Amabile, 1990; Csikszentmihalyi, 1990; Woodman & Schoenfeldt, 1989).

Much of current relational thinking about the environment and creativity has come from researchers and theorists on organizational behavior (Ekvall & Ryhammar, 1999; James et al., 1999; West & Farr, 1990; Woodman, Sawyer, & Griffin, 1993). Organizational variables that influence creativity have been examined as they relate to families, schools, societies, and work organizations. This literature was new to me, and rather fascinating. All individuals are part of these family and community organizations. As such, all individuals are influenced by both the opportunities and constraints of these organizations as they relate to creativity. This literature on organizational creativity helps us think of creativity not only as it relates to an individual within his or her immediate environment but also as it relates to an individual within a larger social system.

The opportunities and constraints of organizational behavior that affect the creativity of each one of us can be readily identified. In the research that I carried out with Virginia Dickie (Hasselkus & Dickie, 1994), several participant occupational therapists in the study told stories of especially dissatisfying experiences of practice that illustrated organizational climates that did not support creativity. Lack of support from administrators, family members, or other staff for new ideas, a sense of having "no control" over decision-making about new options, and resistance to change from supervisors appeared in the stories.

Remember the therapist quoted in Chapter 2 who described her efforts to implement an innovative plan for changing the dining program in a long-term care facility. She was obviously a therapist who could think "outside the box," but her ideas met with strong administrative resistance. In the dining room story, the constraints and opportunities for creativity in an organizational environment were evident. Support from the director of nursing was at first encouraging. The therapist's creativity was not allowed to flourish beyond this point, however; she reported running into strong opposition to her idea from the administrator whom she saw as "powerful" and in control. Ultimately, after several other incidents, the therapist felt that nothing could be accomplished by pursuing her ideas any further; the situation was a "dead end." She ended up voluntarily leaving.

## Creativity From Within—Thinking and Problem Solving

In contrast to our focus thus far on the physical and social environments as they enhance or constrain creativity, we can, of course, also look within the individual for the gestation of creativity. There are theorists who focus primarily, if not solely, on the cognitive processes of thinking and problem solving for their definitions and descriptions of creative phenomena (de Bono, 1970; Guilford, 1950; Milgram, 1990; Torrance, 1988). How creativity arises from such cognitive processes has been described in several different ways; for example, as divergent thinking (Guilford), lateral thinking (de Bono), and ideational fluency (Torrance). Cognitive processes such as these represent *breadth* of thinking or what Getzels and Csikszentmihalyi (1976) called *delay of closure*; they reflect abilities to generate wide-ranging ideas that are drawn from real-world categories of experience and knowledge (Seitz, 1997). For example, in de Bono's concept of lateral thinking, the mind is described as a "patternmaking system" (1970, p. 27); as such, within the mind, information gets sorted out and organizes itself into patterns. Lateral thinking is concerned with facilitating new patterns; "*The most basic principle of lateral thinking is that any particular way*

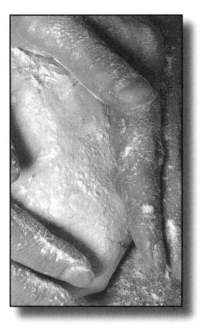

*of looking at things is only one from among many other possible ways.* Lateral thinking is concerned with exploring these other ways by restructuring and rearranging the information that is available" (p. 63, emphasis added).

de Bono (1970) and others (Cameron, 1992; Engelman, 2000, 2005; Goff, 1997; Siau, 1999) spoke of strategies and occupations that one can use to help foster creativity; these strategies assist a person to challenge assumptions, practice the generation of alternative ways of looking at things, restructure patterns, and suspend judgment. In her study on quilting, Dickie (2004) came to the conclusion that the structure and conventional patterns provided at the beginning of a quilt-making project functioned as a stimulus for creative thinking during the actual making of the quilt; instead of acting as a constraint, the quilt patterns actually "afford the opportunity for quilt makers to be creative" (p. 53). According to Cameron, in the use of such strategies or occupations, a person is creating new pathways "through which the creative forces can operate" (p. xiii).

Brainstorming is another strategy for facilitating divergent thinking. In Engelman's (2000) delightful article about her creativity activities with the Belleville Ladies, a group of older women she met with for 6 years at a senior center in rural Wisconsin, she described a brainstorming activity planned around the statement, "Things I'm *not* going to do now that I'm over 70." After some rather traditional responses to the statement (such as scrub the floor on my hands and knees, wear high heels, make a big dinner for my family), the women ventured into more daring territory, or as Engelman said, they "delighted themselves with not-so-typical ideas such as: go anywhere if I don't want to, keep my mouth shut, … feel I have to wash the dishes at night … have a man friend … be so concerned with what others think, restrain myself from spitting" (p. 22). I am more than curious about what prompted that last idea—to let the spit fly! The author described the brainstorming activity as an opportunity for the women to stretch their thinking and to be spontaneous and assertive. This small article plus Engelman's book titled *Aerobics of the Mind* (2005) are goldmines for ideas for facilitating creativity in people who are older.

Other researchers (Cropley, 1992; Goff, 1997; Ruscio & Amabile, 1999; Torrance & Safter, 1990) have focused their attention on ways to break down cognitive barriers to creative thinking in school settings, examining relationships between various instructional styles and student creativity, and proposing strategies to encourage divergent thinking. Being "stuck" in only certain ways of thinking has been variously called functional fixity, cognitive set, and cognitive bias (Cupchik, 1999; Ruscio & Amabile); all such barriers may prevent people from seeing their world in new and unconventional ways or from acknowledging more than one kind of solution to a particular problem.

## *Creativity From Within—Nuances and Metaphors*

Creativity may also be thought of as arising from inner sensitivities and states of consciousness. Briggs (1990) has proposed that early sensitivity to nuances, such as sensitivity to subtle meanings in events (not seen by all people), is what distinguishes creative individuals from those who are not creative. Perhaps the therapist in the dining room story was sensitive to the nuances of the dining room experience for the residents of the nursing home in a way that the administrator was not. She spoke of the lack of dignity present in the current system and her wish to bring about more of a sense of community. Such concerns may reflect subtle meanings of the dining program, apparent to the occupational therapist but not to the administrator.

Seitz (1997) argued that *metaphoric* understanding is the heart of creativity. Seitz defines metaphor as "the ability to link disparate perceptual, affective, and conceptual domains" (p. 347). One metaphor for creativity, cited earlier, links the psychological and physical domains of everyday life—that is, creativity described as the ability to "think outside the box." In this metaphor, the shape of a box is linked to thinking; that is, physical properties are assigned to a mental activity; a physical object is linked to an abstraction. Seitz said, "Metaphor is central to creativity because it involves the ability to detect unity in variety" (p. 348). Metaphors are statements of unity that pull together the multifaceted aspects of complex situations.

Becker (1997) referred to metaphors as important precursors to change; "Through metaphor people are able to reframe the inexplicable and reorganize their lives" (p. 65). Metaphors help people find new meanings in familiar situations.

In some ways, the concept of metaphor as the heart of creativity is the opposite of the concepts of divergent thinking or lateral thinking; whereas metaphors express commonalities and a sense of wholeness and unity across differences, sort of a gestalt, divergent thinking seeks to separate out the many different elements of a domain and to express them in as broad a range of different options as possible. Metaphor pulls elements together, encapsulates meanings across widely disparate domains; divergent thinking opens out, wider and wider, leading to more and more possibilities. They are indeed very different concepts of creativity.

## ARISING FROM CHAOS

"One must still have chaos in oneself to be able to give birth to a dancing star" (Nietzsche, from *Thus Spoke Zarathustra*, 1973). This oft-quoted line from the 19th-century philosopher Friedrich Nietzsche beautifully expresses the idea of chaos as the birthplace of creativity (i.e., the birthplace of "a dancing star"). Nietzsche's sentiment reflects the principles of chaos as the origin for creativity.

*Chaos* and *chaos theory* are terms that appear periodically in any search of the literature on creativity. Chaos theory focuses on the examination of discontinuities in life systems and the emergence of new states of being (Zausner, 1998). A system in a state of chaos is far from equilibrium, it is unstable; in such a state, multiple options become available and the system can veer off into totally new directions or fundamentally reorganize itself. One can see creativity elements of inspiration, breaking cognitive sets, and new pattern formation in the concept of chaos.

The behavior of a system in chaos is intrinsically unpredictable. Kellert (1993) referred to the unpredictability of the system as the "crucial scientific characteristic" of chaos theory (p. x). The unpredictability of a chaotic system results from a further feature known as *sensitive dependence on initial conditions* (Kellert; Smith, 1998). How a system changes over time and circumstances is exquisitely sensitive to its initial conditions. Because we can never wholly and entirely know its initial conditions, and because the tiniest errors or mistakes or omissions regarding the initial conditions will become tremendously magnified in short time, we can never wholly predict what changes are going to take place. Small errors do not stay small; small errors lead to unpredictable but large changes.

Kellert (1993) used human history to illustrate these principles of chaos theory. One may detect broad patterns in the rise and fall of civilizations across the ages, but events never repeat themselves exactly. Further, history books are full of examples of "small events that led to momentous and long-lasting changes in the course of human affairs" (p. 5). As just one example, one might think of the 1972 Watergate break-in, subsequent investigations and hearings, and ultimate resignation of Richard Nixon from the presidency of the United States. As another example, the standard 8.5 by 11-inch paper size used in the United States originated with the Remington typewriter company in conjunction with decisions regarding the width of the typewriter roller and keyboard; to think of the enormous consequences of the size of that paper on the design of all typewriters, envelopes, three-ring binders, file drawers, copy machines, scanners, computer printers, computer commands, font sizes, etc., is mind-boggling.

In this age of ever-evolving technology, new dimensions of chaos and chaotic solutions are being generated. *Fractals* are complicated computer-generated images that represent unstable and unpredictable chaotic solutions to mathematical equations. Fractals offer a way to visualize chaos in our world. Wheatley (1999) said that fractals reveal "the partnering of chaos and order" in our world (p. 128) and that they occur naturally all around us (e.g., in branching trees, grasses, clouds). Fractals are chaotic but bounded; they never settle down to a fixed value or even to a repeating pattern, but neither do they fly off into infinity. These beautiful and mysterious objects can be viewed in full color at the following Web site: http://sprott.physics.wisc.edu/fractals.htm (accessed October 5, 2010).

Like chaos theory and Cohen's (2000) creativity with a little c, the therapist's proposed changes in the dining room held the possibility for demonstrating the power of small changes to bring about larger ones—for a simple rearrangement of people and the eating environment to bring about the creation of community and the reestablishment of dignity for individuals. Unlike chaos theory, however, the therapist was convinced that she could *predict* events that would follow her changes; perhaps the administrator foresaw outcomes more like those of a system in chaos—instability and many *unpredictable* elements including potential large changes that would cause great difficulties from a management standpoint. As Becker (1997) said, orderliness and predictability are part of the American cultural ideology; unpredictability is unsettling. Ideas for new and novel actions hold an inherent element of risk and unpredictability that may or may not be considered acceptable by those individuals who are within the sphere of influence.

# CREATIVITY AND HEALTH

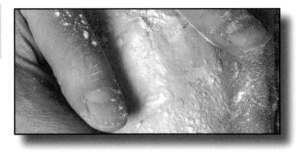

The relationship of creativity to health and well-being, as proposed in the literature, is fascinating. Runco and Richards (1997) stated simply that everyday creativity is good for one's health.

> The everyday practice of originality may enhance physical as well as psychological well-being. ... To do, to grow, to risk, to change, to know oneself, and the world about us—and also to dare to know what one does *not* know—can be healthy and good, and even life-giving. (p. x)

Blanche (2007) referred to the creative process as "a powerful vehicle for expressing one's authentic self" (p. 26). And Dickie (2004) discussed beliefs in the profession that creativity stems from a biological need in humans, that it is a natural quality of life, and that this quality needs to be fostered and restored when it is threatened. She refers to this fundamental human need as a "creative imperative" (p. 55).

Taking it one step further, Bodine (1999) and Phillips (1999) spoke of creativity as a healing force; Bodine said, "Creativity is one of the most valuable tools we have to aid us in our healing process" (p. 120) and Phillips stated, "The act of creating is a healing gesture, as sacred as prayer, as essential to the spirit as food to the body" (p. 126). The profession of art therapy is strongly devoted to this view of creativity, with a particular emphasis on psychoanalytic healing processes (Keyes, 1983).

Conversely, Zausner (1998) wrote that, for some, creativity is triggered by episodes of severe or prolonged ill health; this view is one of creativity that arises from illness, rather than or in addition to creativity as a healing force to overcome illness. As Zausner stated, "When viewed as a period of transformative chaos, physical illness, although generally seen as negative, may also have positive aspects" (p. 22).

And finally, let us not forget that creativity has a dark side as well as a bright side. Expressions of creativity are phenomena that disregard or challenge established ways of thinking and behaving (Brower, 1999); thus, by definition, creativity may be viewed as a form of rebellion. Sometimes these creative challenges take forms that are unacceptable to society.

## Everyday Creativity and Health

Allen (1995) said, "The gift of creativity is within each of us waiting to unfold" (xvi). Everyday creativity can be a very strong experience. We have all known the lift of spirit that comes when we experience moments of creativity. For me, when I have an idea that seems somehow special and inspired, I feel wonderful and I find myself eager to share my creative moment with someone. I like what Annie Dillard said of such a moment—"It is a glowing thing, a blurred thing of beauty" (1989, p. 56). Besides sharing the "glowing thing," I want to continue to "work" with the idea while it is "hot." I get very "revved up"; I cannot sleep; I cannot turn off my thinking; I am driven to getting a firmer hold on the idea, almost as though I feel the need to capture it right away or risk losing the idea forever.

Cameron (1992) would refer to the experience of creativity that I have just described as "spiritual electricity" (p. 1). In Cameron's book, *The Artist's Way*, the author's primary message is that life itself is pure creative energy. Further, this creative energy dwells within each one of us. If we deny or refuse to use our creativity, we are taking an action that runs counter to our true nature. To Cameron, creativity is our *raison d'etre*; her book details a spiritual process whereby we may experience "creative recovery" (p. 5), thereby becoming a more fully functioning and more conscious being in the world.

As far as I can determine, creativity of everyday life is a largely unresearched topic. An early work by Nicholls (1972) investigated everyday creativity as a trait, present in a variable amount in all human beings. Others, since Nicholls, have approached the concept of everyday creativity from specific orientations such as mental health (Richards et al., 1997), cognition (Necka, 1986), personality and intelligence (Barron & Harrington, 1981), and mental functioning (Cropley, 1997). Yet, all of these attempts to understand and define everyday creativity seem woefully inadequate, dry as bones. Somehow, finding creativity's "lift of spirit" or "spiritual electricity" in theories of cognition and personality is difficult.

To me, everyday creativity can be manifested in any ordinary aspect of our day-to-day lives—that tasty casserole concocted from leftovers from dinner last night, the wide-ranging ideas expressed in discussion at work, the eye-catching letter to the editor composed for the newspaper, the "just right" words used to comfort an anguished friend, the impulsive purchase of a second-hand oriental rug at a garage sale to decorate the office, the "lullaby" made up to calm the crying baby, the funky wallpaper picked out for the newly remodeled kitchen. These are the aspects of our ordinary days that give us a special sense of "life." These are creative moments "filled with spirit" (Cassou, 1999, p. 3), done for their own sake, free.

Myers (1999) said, "In creating we bring forth life, and with life comes health" (p. xvi). Having our creativity squelched, an experience probably most of us have had at one time or another, is painful. The spirit of the moment is instantly dispelled; the sense of freedom and spontaneity is lost. I know I have at times been guilty of squelching enthusiastic graduate students when they come forth with fresh ideas about the research they are conducting—ideas that have seemed unrealistic or naïve or undeveloped to my "more experienced" eye. Afterwards, I think, "How could I have done that?" In my immediate squelching of their ideas, I have taken away all the freedom and spirit and life of the moment. I know in my heart that such reactions are no way to mentor a student, and I vow to try to do better next time.

In occupational therapy, we as therapists have unending opportunities for creative moments in our work. Every client whom we see is unique; every treatment plan we develop and carry out is unique; every time we engage in clinical reasoning, we are using our creative energies to make sense out of the many elements of each new clinical situation. Often these creative moments are what give us so much satisfaction in our careers. They support our work life and our own health in that work life.

In therapy, we focus our energies and attention on the everyday occupations of the people with whom we work. Because of our emphasis on the ordinary, in a world of medical care (a world that is in every other way *not* ordinary), we, in occupational therapy, must depend on a highly improvisational style of being therapists (Mattingly, 1998). In our profession, we are rarely protocol driven; the therapy that we offer is created on the spot.

In her story of a very satisfying experience in practice (Hasselkus & Dickie, 1994), a therapist described her work with a young man who fell off a roof the week before he was to enter medical school, fracturing both of his arms "pretty seriously." The therapist's sense of satisfaction found in the creative elements of her therapy with the man is evident in the following narrative:

> He was casted, both arms were casted in a position where his elbows were in flexion and he really could do nothing for himself. He had the option to wait, postponing med school for a year, or learning how to adapt and do things for himself. And so with creative creating, I guess, we spent a lot of time and adapted everything from the fork, the spoon, the toothbrush, something for him to wipe himself with, and came up with techniques for just about anything you can think of that you needed to do. He ended up going to med school, and the only thing he couldn't do for himself was completely shower, he needed someone to help him get the baggies on his arms so he wouldn't get the casts wet. That stands out as something that really made a difference in somebody's life immediately. And it was really an OT-type thing to be able to be creative and design equipment.

For some of us, the creative dimension of the profession is one of its main attractions. As illustrated in the story above, the practice of occupational therapy is a far cry from carrying out recipe-like protocols or following through on detailed orders for prescribed treatment. The everydayness of the practice is poignantly evident in the references to the fork and the toothbrush and "something for him to wipe himself with." The therapist herself refers to her therapy as "creative creating" and says that what she was able to do "really made a difference in somebody's life immediately." The young man was able to go to med school, and that, to the therapist, was the very satisfying outcome of what she did—her spiritual electricity.

## Creativity as a Healing Force

"Creativity has the power to alter the darkness in our lives, whether we paint with it, draw with it, write with it, sing with it, work or play with it, or even just think with it" (Cohen, 2000, p. 200). The concept of creativity as a healing force, able to "alter the darkness in our lives," occurs over and over again in the literature. Healing powers are attributed to poem making, storytelling, photography, journal writing, painting, dance, and music. Alternatively, the healing power of creativity can also be associated with the more mundane and ordinary occupations of our day-to-day living. Bodine (1999) described the creativity of everyday life as a "happy energy" (p. 124) and attributed "a certain magic" to its healing power (p. 125).

I was surprised when I reviewed the several bodies of literature for this chapter to find that the foundations of art therapy, begun in the late 1950s, continue to this day to be drawn almost entirely from psychotherapy (see, for example, Case & Dalley, 1992; Cohen, 1971; Keyes, 1983; Levy, 1995; Malchiodi, 1998). Creativity linked to other psychotherapeutic clinical contexts is also strongly present in the literature, such as in the often-cited book edited by Runco and Richards (1997); individual chapters (and chapter titles) highlight topics such as alcoholism, manic depression, mood disorders, psychopathology, and ego functioning. The gerontology literature abounds in reports of the positive effects of creative activities on the potentially debilitating conditions of old age; for example, Osgood, Meyers, and Orchowsky (1990) reported on the impact of creative dance on the life satisfaction of older adults; Hanser (1990) published results of a music therapy program for depressed older adults in the community; and Peck (1989) shared the health-promoting responses of the nursing home residents who participated in her poetry writing groups.

Allen (1995) lamented this transformation of art into a "treatment modality" composed of prescribed goals and outcomes and predetermined interpretations (p. xvi). Allen's thoughts illustrate a tension that exists between those who think of art as a medium for assessment and treatment in clinical settings and those who think of art as the medium by which we can come to know and to be our authentic selves. To Allen, the art-making of art therapy is a "sanitized, soulless version of art" (p. xvi) that is administered to others and that requires the interpretation of trained professionals. Alternatively, she considered authentic art making as a "key to soul … a crucial and sustaining part of life" (p. xix). In the profession of occupational therapy, we have parallel tensions associated with the concept of occupation; we try to be a bridge between its use and meaning in the clinical world *and* its meaning and relationship to well-being in the nonmedical arenas of day-to-day life.

My natural inclination is to turn toward the literature that speaks to the everyday healing experience of creativity. I believe that power *can* exist in the prescribed use of art for psychoanalysis and healing. But the power of creativity as a healing force exists more strongly for me in the ordinary day-to-day experiences of creativity with which we are all familiar.

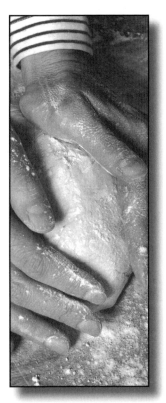

In Mattingly's (1998) narrative framework, the ritual healing of occupational therapy requires the therapist to make of therapy a social drama in which the therapist and patient create together events that hold healing power. She describes occupational therapy as "a 'ritual of the everyday' played out in the clinical world" (p. 165). It is precisely through our creative rituals "of the everyday" that we strive to bring healing to the people with whom we work.

The therapist in the previous story about the medical student felt especially satisfied with her work with this client; it seems obvious that the sense of having been creative in her therapy contributed strongly to her sense of satisfaction. But what about the medical student, himself? What was his part in this "social drama"? Did he, too, have a creative experience and benefit from the healing potential that such experiences offer?

These are questions that speak to the importance of the concept of client-centered practice. If creativity has healing power, then ought not therapists consider their clients' potential creativity as they plan therapy—purposely building in opportunities for clients to experience their own creativity as part of the therapy process? Dickie (2004) said that we should do exactly that; we need to "find ways of supporting individuals to try creativity" (p. 56). A small number of programs that illustrate such efforts are reported in our professional literature (for example, Reynold's [2003] research on using artistic occupation to help forge positive identities in women with chronic illness; Ramugondo's [2004] work on play and playfulness as health-giving occupations in children with HIV/AIDS in South Africa; and the work of Ciukaj, Suarez-Balcazar, & Field [2009] on creative drama and children with disabilities). Reynolds and Prior (2006) studied the experience of creative occupation among women living with cancer, finding that the women's engagement in visual art-making "helped to banish intrusive thoughts about cancer, provided valued experiences of mastery and control and encouraged the participants to engage in positive journeys into the unknown, thereby alleviating some of the stress of cancer" (p. 255).

Kitwood and Bredin (1992) have proposed creativity as one of several indicators of relative well-being in persons with dementia; surely, then, providing the opportunity for such a client to experience creativity is one therapeutic way to use occupation in dementia care. In occupational therapy, as is perhaps not the case in any other health field, the potential for clients to experience their own creativity is ever present. The satisfaction and sense of well-being that we as therapists experience from working creatively can also be present for the patients and clients with whom we work.

In our research on satisfying and dissatisfying experiences in occupational therapy (Hasselkus & Dickie, 1994), we heard some stories in which the therapist spoke with special joy of the client's contributions to the therapy: "We did a lot of neat adaptive equipment and he actually helped to design some of his own equipment. … I think that

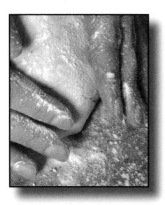

is what made it really fun, was that he was also taking a real active part in his therapy." Yet, as in this case, the therapist seemed to feel satisfaction from the motivation and commitment represented by the client's involvement and enjoyment in the experience of working together, but she did not seem to recognize the healing potential of the client's creative involvement in the therapy. I would agree with Perrin (2001) and suggest that the client's creativity is an untapped, or at least unrecognized, source of the healing and well-being that can result from therapy and that the occupational core of occupational therapy offers a very rich resource for creative opportunities in a patient's life.

## From Illness Comes Creativity

As we now know, chaos theory addresses discontinuities, loss of equilibrium, and the emergence of new states of being (Zausner, 1998). The word *chaos* has also been used as a metaphor for illness. Becker (1997) said, "When their health is suddenly disrupted, people are thrown into chaos. … People experience the time before their illness and its aftermath as two separate realities. This perception of a dual reality—of the known world (the recent past) and the 'bad dream' (the present)—constitutes chaos" (p. 37). Illness disrupts the orderliness of life; "when the body is assaulted by a serious illness, one's sense of wholeness, on which a sense of order rides, disintegrates" (p. 39).

Zausner (1998) referred to illness as "creative chaos" (p. 21) and characterized it as a time of transition to a new life stage and the production of new art. He discusses a number of artists, who, for example, experienced serious illness in their early lives; these periods of illness seemed to serve as turning points that led to subsequent surges of creative activity. Matisse, for example (see Flam, 1986), was a young man recovering from appendicitis when he became acquainted with art supplies; he is quoted as saying that the moment the box of colors was in his hands, he had the feeling that his life was laid out before him. During his adulthood, the Spanish artist Goya had an infection that left him deaf; after this period of illness, his paintings changed, became darker and more psychologically detailed (Perez Sanchez & Sayre, 1989). As Zausner said, "The drive to produce art despite physical impediments is what may transform a potential disorder into a creative chaos. As chaos contains the seeds of the new order, so may illness contain the seeds of the new artist and the new art" (p. 27). In this way, Zausner portrayed illness as a period of "transformative chaos" (p. 22).

The concept of illness as a progenitor of creativity is, in many ways, the direct opposite of the previously discussed theme of creativity as healer. In the previous theme, creativity is viewed as a potential power in our lives that can be used to heal and dispel illness; in creativity as healer, illness is negative, something to be gotten rid of, a disruption in the orderly narrative of one's life. In contrast, when thought of as sources of *creativity* instead of disruption, illnesses in one's life become honored states of being. In this view of illness, we recognize that a sickness throws an individual into a state of disequilibrium, but we also recognize that this state of disequilibrium is a potential state of creative chaos. A person who is experiencing a serious or prolonged illness may fundamentally reorganize him- or herself, producing a new, transformed order and state of being.

But many of these examples are of eminent creativity, not everyday creativity. Closer to the intended focus of this chapter are the small, everyday moments of creativity that emanate from the adversities of life, including illnesses, on a daily basis. In Cohen's book on creativity in aging (2000), he told the charming story of an interview with George Burns when the comedian was 97 years old. In the interview, Burns shared with Cohen the fact that he had recently developed back pain and was concerned that it would interfere with his comic routines. Some colleagues had counseled him to sit down while he did his routines, but Burns, at first, thought this would not work well; after all, he said (tongue in cheek), all his life he had been "a stand-up comic." Eventually he tried sitting during his routine and found, to his surprise, that it had no negative effect on his performance. As for future adaptations, he said, with a smile, "… if necessary, I'll become a lie-down comic" (p. 175).

This story represents, to me, the essence of everyday creativity in the presence of illness or adversity. Burns' change to sitting during his comic routines represented a shift in the way he organized and thought of himself as a comedian, and in his way of *being* a comedian. This was a shift that occurred only with a great deal of concern about whether or not he would still be the comedian he had always been. Once he had made the change, he incorporated it into his life narrative as a source for jokes, and not only jokes about his current state of affairs but even jokes that spoke to possibly more dramatic changes in the future. Jokes were this man's way of life, a huge part of George Burns' identity; what had, at first, appeared as a threat of disorder and "chaos" in his life (having to sit down to do his routines) turned out not to be a threat after all but, instead, was a change that contributed to new thinking and new ways to experience his comedian-self. The temporary state of disequilibrium occasioned by his back pain led to a new way of *being* in his world of comedy.

Cohen (2000) believed that adversity "serves as a prompt for innovative thinking in that we instinctively seek relief from it" (p. 176). Perhaps much of the practice of occupational therapy could be characterized as relying on creativity to offer relief in the face of adversity. Clients come to us because of some form of illness or adversity; we endeavor to come up with creative ways to bring relief from that adversity. The character of the adversity itself is a strong driving force that guides our creativity.

## The Dark Side of Creativity

I stated earlier that one way to consider creativity is as a form of rebellion (Brower, 1999). The communication of new ideas to the "others" in our world exposes our inner selves to the outside world. New ideas serve as a strong expression of the self of the person who offers them. To be effective, a person who rebels must be willing to pay the price of the rebellion. Brower stated, "All rebellion, ultimately, is a rebellion of the self" (p. 9).

To some extent, a natural tension exists in all cultures among the phenomena of deviance, creativity, and conformity. In the United States, where we tend to be particularly sensitive to anything that smacks of censorship, we struggle with where to draw the line between pornography and art, between exploitation and realism, between obscenity and frank expression, between good and bad nonconformity. What one person claims is creative, another may label as deviant or trash. The word *deviant* harbors the notion of intentionality (rebellion) in Western culture and implies a violation of values or rules; as an attribute, deviance is largely linked to the behavior of adults. Yet Waksler (1987), in her study of the behaviors of kindergarteners, demonstrated how teachers often label the behaviors of children as deviant. How far outside the boundaries of usual expectations the behaviors or products lie, and just what the consequences of these violated societal values are, determine the label that is used. As Brower said, "Creativity and deviance are in many ways synonymous" (1999, p. 3). Is it creative or deviant to dye one's hair a brilliant blue? Is it creative or deviant to convert one's front lawn into a natural prairie? Is it creative or deviant to figure out a foolproof way to cheat on an exam without getting caught? Is it creative or deviant to suggest that all nursing home residents dine in the same room?

Cropley (1973) has suggested that social systems are like a continuum of concentric rings, each reflecting a level of social sanctions on behaviors. At the core of the rings is behavior that is strictly forbidden, taboo, in any and all circumstances; sexual relationships between a parent and a son or daughter might constitute such a taboo behavior.

The next ring comprises behaviors that are socially unacceptable or barely acceptable and that meet with strong disapproval. Surrounding this ring is a third that comprises behaviors that are somewhat acceptable but that meet with slight disapproval. These levels of disapproval are not problematic in and of themselves; it goes without saying that groups of people need guidelines and rules and laws by which to govern collective and individual behaviors. However, as Cropley stated more recently, "The problem from the point of view of creativity ... is that rules may go far beyond what is needed for peaceful coexistence, and may become rigid and self-perpetuating" (1997, p. 238). Creative people, who are by nature unconventional, may become marginalized when the rules are rigid.

To address the apparent paradox of being able to experience unconventionality without being marginalized, Cropley (1997) suggested the following: "... creativity requires the capacity to diverge from the norm, but simultaneously to function within the society's rules" (p. 239). Whether or not one can do that, however, and still be true to one's self and one's principles, is a formidable question.

## TO THE DANCING STAR

Creativity arises from our physical and social worlds and from the sensitivities and thinking processes of our inner selves. Creativity is Nietzsche's "dancing star" of our lives. Many believe that the experience of everyday creativity supports health and well-being.

In occupational therapy, opportunities to experience everyday creativity are ever-present—for both the therapist and for the client. The health-promoting potential found in the experience of creativity deserves more attention. As Bindeman (1998) has said, creativity is a "significant and uniquely human experience" (p. 69). May we increasingly recognize its presence in the lives of all of us and its contribution to our health and well-being.

## REFERENCES

Allen, P. B. (1995). *Art is a way of knowing*. Boston, MA: Shambhala Publications.

Amabile, T. M. (1990). Within you, without you: The social psychology of creativity, and beyond. In M. A. Runco & R. S. Albert (Eds.), *Theories of creativity* (pp. 61-91). Newbury Park, CA: Sage.

Barron, F. X., & Harrington, D. M. (1981). Creativity, intelligence and personality. *Annual Review of Psychology, 32,* 439-476.

Becker, G. (1997). *Disrupted lives: How people create meaning in a chaotic world*. Berkeley, CA: University of California Press.

Bindeman, S. (1998). Echoes of silence: A phenomenological study of the creative process. *Creativity Research Journal, 11,* 69-77.

Blanche, E. I. (2007). The expression of creativity through occupation. *Journal of Occupational Science, 14,* 21-29.

Bodine, E. (1999). The healing power of creativity. In T. P. Myers (Ed.), *The soul of creativity: Insights into the creative process* (pp. 120-125). Novato, CA: New World Library.

Briggs, J. (1990). *Fire in the crucible*. Los Angeles, CA: Tarcher.

Brower, R. (1999). Dangerous minds: Eminently creative people who spent time in jail. *Creativity Research Journal, 12,* 3-13.

Cameron, J. (1992). *The artist's way: A spiritual path to higher creativity*. New York, NY: Jeremy P. Tarcher/Putnam.

Case, C., & Dalley, T. (1992). *Handbook of art therapy*. New York, NY: Routledge.

Cassou, M. (1999). Inside the heartbeat of creation. In T. P. Myers (Ed.), *The soul of creativity: Insights into the creative process* (pp. 2-6). Novato, CA: New World Library.

Ciukaj, M., Suarez-Balcazar, Y., & Field, S. B. (2009). Incorporating creative drama into the lives of children with disabilities. *OT Practice*.

Cohen, F. W. (1971). *Mark and the paint brush*. Austin, TX: Hogg Foundation for Mental Health, University of Texas.

Cohen, G. D. (2000). *The creative age: Awakening human potential in the second half of life*. New York: Avon Books.

Cropley, A. J. (1973). Creativity and culture. *Educational Trends, 8,* 19-27.

Cropley, A. J. (1992). *More ways than one: Fostering creativity*. Norwood, NJ: Ablex.

Cropley, A. J. (1997). Creativity and mental health in everyday life. In M. A. Runco & R. Richards (Eds.), *Eminent creativity, everyday creativity, and health* (pp. 231-246). Greenwich, CT: Ablex.

Csikszentmihalyi, M. (1990). The domain of creativity. In M. A. Runco, & R. S. Albert (Eds.), *Theories of creativity* (pp. 190-212). Newbury Park, CA: Sage.

Cupchik, G. C. (1999). The thinking-I and the being-I in psychology of the arts. *Creative Research Journal, 12,* 165-173.

de Bono, E. (1970). *Lateral thinking: Creativity step by step*. New York, NY: Harper & Row.

Dickie, V. A. (2004). From drunkard's path to Kansas cyclones: Discovering creativity inside the blocks. *Journal of Occupational Science, 11,* 51-57.

Dillard, A. (1989). *The writing life*. New York, NY: Harper & Row.

Ekvall, G., & Ryhammar, L. (1999). The creative climate: Its determinants and effects at a Swedish university. *Creativity Research Journal, 12,* 303-310.

Engelman, M. (2000). Here's to the Belleville ladies: Creativity in aging. *Activities, Adaptation & Aging, 24*(4), 19-26.

Engelman, M. (2005). *Aerobics of the mind*. State College, PA: Venture Publishing.

Feldhusen, J. F., & Goh, B. E. (1995). Assessing and accessing creativity: An integrative review of theory, research and development. *Creativity Research Journal, 8,* 231-247.

Flam, J. (1986). *Matisse. The man and his art*. Ithaca, NY: Cornell University Press.

Getzels, J. W., & Csikszentmihalyi, M. (1976). *The creative vision: A longitudinal study of problem finding in art*. New York, NY: Wiley.

Goff, K. (1997). *Everyday creativity*. Stillwater, OK: Little Ox Books.

Guilford, J. P. (1950). Creativity. *American Psychologist, 5,* 444 454.

Hanser, S. B. (1990). A music therapy strategy for depressed older adults in the community. *Journal of Applied Gerontology, 9,* 283-298.

Harrington, D. M. (1990). The ecology of human creativity: A psychological perspective. In M. A. Runco, & R. S. Albert (Eds.), *Theories of creativity* (pp. 143-169). Newbury Park, CA: Sage.

Hasselkus, B. R., & Dickie, V. A. (1994). Doing occupational therapy: Dimensions of satisfaction and dissatisfaction. *American Journal of Occupational Therapy, 48,* 145-154.

James, K., Clark, K., & Cropanzano, R. (1999). Positive and negative creativity in groups, institutions, and organizations: A model and theoretical extension. *Creativity Research Journal, 12,* 211-226.

Kellert, S. H. (1993). *In the wake of chaos: Unpredictable order in dynamical systems*. Chicago, IL: The University of Chicago Press.

Keyes, M. F. (1983). *Inward journey: Art as therapy*. LaSalle, IL: Open Court.

Kitwood, T., & Bredin, K. (1992). Towards a theory of dementia care: Personhood and well-being. *Aging and Society, 12*, 269-287.

Levy, F. J. (1995). *Dance and other expressive art therapies*. New York, NY: Routledge.

Mace, M. A. (1997). Toward an understanding of creativity through a qualitative appraisal of contemporary art making. *Creativity Research Journal, 10*, 265-278.

Malchiodi, C. A. (1998). *Understanding children's drawings*. New York, NY: Guilford.

Mattingly, C. (1998). *Healing dramas and clinical plots: The narrative structure of experience*. Cambridge, UK: Cambridge University Press.

McNiff, S. (1998). *Trust the process: An artist's guide to letting go*. Boston, MA: Shambhala Publications.

Milgram, R. M. (1990). Creativity: An idea whose time has come and gone? In M. A. Runco & R. S. Albert (Eds.), *Theories of creativity* (pp. 215-233). Newbury Park, CA: Sage.

Myers, T. P. (1999). *The soul of creativity: Insights into the creative process*. Novato, CA: New World Library.

Necka, E. (1986). On the nature of creative talent. In A. J. Cropley, K. K. Urban, H. Wagner, & W. H. Wieczerkowski (Eds.), *Giftedness: A continuing worldwide challenge* (pp. 131-140). New York, NY: Trillium.

Nicholls, J. G. (1972). Creativity in the person who will never produce anything original or useful: The concept of creativity as a normally distributed trait. *American Psychologist, 27*, 717-727.

Nietzsche, F. W. (1973). Thus spoke Zarathustra. In W. Kaufman (Ed. & Trans.), *The portable Nietzsche* (pp. 103-439). New York, NY: Viking Press.

Osgood, N. J., Meyers, B. S., & Orchowsky, S. (1990). The impact of creative dance and movement training on the life satisfaction of older adults: An exploratory study. *Journal of Applied Gerontology, 9*, 255-265.

Peck, C. F. (1989). *From deep within*. New York, NY: Haworth Press.

Peloquin, S. M. (1997). The spiritual depth of occupation: Making worlds and making lives. *American Journal of Occupational Therapy, 51*, 167-168.

Perez Sanchez, A. E., & Sayre, E. A. (1989). *Goya and the spirit of enlightenment*. Boston, MA: Little Brown.

Perrin, T. (2001). Don't despise the fluffy bunny: A reflection from practice. *British Journal of Occupational Therapy, 64*, 129-134.

Phillips. J. (1999). Creativity: The healing journey inward. In T. P. Myers (Ed.), *The soul of creativity: Insights into the creative process* (pp. 126-132). Novato, CA: New World Library.

Ramugondo, E. L. (2004). Play and playfulness: Children living with HIV/AIDS. In R. Watson & L. Swartz (Eds.), *Transformation through occupation*. London, UK: Whurr Publishers.

Reynolds, F. (2003). Reclaiming a positive identity in chronic illness through artistic occupation. *OTJR: Occupation, Participation and Health, 23*, 118-127.

Reynolds, F., & Prior, S. (2006). Creative adventures and flow in art-making: A qualitative study of women living with cancer. *British Journal of Occupational Therapy, 69*, 255-262.

Richards, R., Kinney, D. K., Lunde, I., Benet, M., & Merzel, A. P. C. (1997). Creativity in manic-depressives, cyclothymes, their normal relatives, and control subjects. In A. Runco & R. Richards (Eds.), *Eminent creativity, everyday creativity, and health* (pp. 119-136). Greenwich, CT: Ablex.

Runco, M. A., & Richards, R. (Eds.). (1997). *Eminent creativity, everyday creativity and health*. Greenwich, CT: Ablex.

Ruscio, A. M., & Amabile, T. M. (1999). Effects of instructional style on problem-solving creativity. *Creativity Research Journal, 12,* 251-266.

SARK. (1999). Make it real. In T. P. Myers (Ed.), *The soul of creativity* (pp. 39-44). Novato, CA: New World Library.

Seitz, J. A. (1997). The development of metaphoric understanding: Implications for a theory of creativity. *Creativity Research Journal, 10,* 347-353.

Siau, K. (1999). Internet, World Wide Web, and creativity. *Journal of Creative Behavior, 33,* 191-201.

Smith, P. (1998). *Explaining chaos.* Cambridge, UK: Cambridge University Press.

Toomey, M. (2003). Creativity: Access to the spirit through occupation. In M. A. McColl (Ed.), *Spirituality and occupational therapy* (pp. 181-192). Canadian Association of Occupational Therapy.

Torrance, F. P. (1988). The nature of creativity as manifest in its testing. In R. G. Sternberg (Ed.), *The nature of creativity: Contemporary perspectives* (pp. 43-75). New York, NY: Cambridge University Press.

Torrance, E. P., & Safter, H. T. (1990). *The incubation model of teaching: Getting beyond aha!* Buffalo, NY: Bearly Limited.

Waksler, F. C. (1987). Dancing when the music is over: A study of deviance in a kindergarten classroom. *Sociological Studies of Child Development, 2,* 139-158.

West, M. A., & Farr, J. L. (1990). *Innovation and creativity at work: Psychological and organizational strategies.* West Sussex, England: Wiley.

Wheatley, M. J. (1999). *Leadership and the new science. Discovering order in a chaotic world* (2nd ed.). San Francisco, CA: Berrett-Koehler Publishers.

Wilcock, A. A. (2006). *An occupational perspective of health* (2nd ed.). Thorofare, NJ: SLACK Incorporated.

Woodman, R. W., Sawyer, J. E., & Griffin, R. W. (1993). Toward a theory of organizational creativity. *Academy of Management Review, 18,* 293-321.

Woodman, R. W., & Schoenfeldt, L. F. (1989). Individual differences in creativity: An interactionist perspective. In J. A. Glover, R. R. Ronning, & C. R. Reynolds (Eds.), *Handbook of creativity* (pp. 77-91). New York, NY: Plenum.

Zausner, T. (1998). When walls become doorways: Creativity, chaos theory, and physical illness. *Creativity Research Journal, 11,* 21-28.

# CHAPTER 10

# OCCUPATION SPEAKS: FINAL THOUGHTS

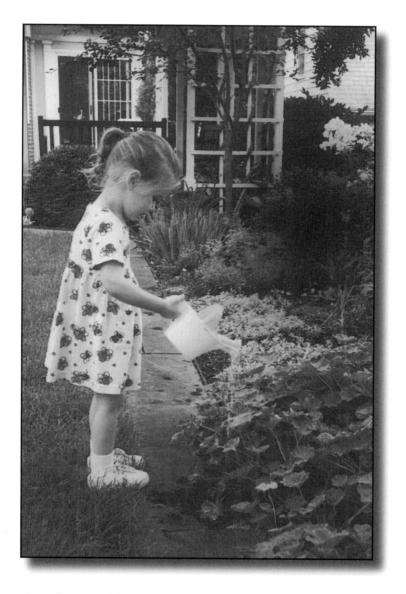

At the still point of the turning world …

Where past and future are gathered. Neither movement from nor towards,

Neither ascent nor decline. Except for the point, the still point,

There would be no dance, and there is only the dance.

T. S. Eliot, lines from "Burnt Norton," *Four Quartets* (1943)

I think these lines from Eliot's poem (Eliot, 1943) capture the essence of what I have been trying to say throughout this book. The meaning of our daily lives lies in the *experiencing* of our daily lives, in the consciousness of the moment, at the still point; there the dance is—and there *is* only the dance.

"The important thing," Susan Lydon said, "is not so much what you knit as what happens to you while you knit it" (1997). It is the *experience*—the dance—of the occupation that is important, not the occupation itself or the outcome. To me, when we pay attention to the experience of occupation, we are able to hear occupation speak. The experience is the interior journey, it is what happens to us while we knit; it is what we find there and how we are transformed. Occupation speaks every day of our lives, all our lives long. We can think of occupation as the vehicle by which we experience our worlds.

In our Western society, there are situations or contexts of life in which experience *is* primary. Think about infancy and young childhood. At those ages, life is *all* about experiencing. For example, when she was 2½ years old, my granddaughter Carolyn loved to water the flowers in the garden. She made countless trips back and forth to the outdoor faucet to refill the sprinkling can. She watered whatever caught her eye. Sometimes she watered the same plant over and over again. It made no difference to her that the plant was drowning! The experience of the sprinkling itself was what she was absorbed in—the flow of the water, the sound of the water, the feel of the water, the sparkling of the water.

But it seems that as we grow older, we begin to attach purpose and goals to all our actions. We expect what we do to end up with a product, either something material like a knitted sweater or an achieved goal such as getting the garden watered. We analyze our actions to determine the reasons behind them, the rationale and purposes. We may get uneasy if we cannot figure out the purpose of our own actions or somebody else's actions. We may get uneasy if there doesn't seem to be anything "productive" about somebody's occupational engagement.

We might even get uneasy with Carolyn's rather random watering efforts and turn our attention to trying to teach her how to tell which plants need watering and which ones do not, and how much water to put on each one, and when to stop already! Perhaps that is the beginning of it all—the beginning of the shift that occurs with a vengeance in later childhood and adulthood, the shift to engagement in occupation for an end, a purpose, rather than engagement in occupation for the sake of the experience itself.

My point is that occupation, in addition to the end products that it yields in the way of completed projects, things, accomplishments, is also comprised of experience. The experiential aspects of occupation are often ignored and devalued in our society; the finished product is what we point to with pride. And yet, to me, the *experience* of the occupation may very well be the most important part.

Our cultural tendency to focus on outcomes instead of experience affects the way we view our occupational therapy practice. This tendency is probably one of the reasons many occupational therapists are not comfortable in certain fields of practice, such as in care for people with dementia or care for people who are dying. Experiencing the moment is what the person with dementia can still do and what the person who is dying can still do. Similarly, therapy with people who have mental

Hasselkus, B. R.
*The Meaning of Everyday Occupation, Second Edition* (pp. 185-188).
© 2011 SLACK Incorporated

illness is work that strongly emphasizes the experiential process of therapy rather than measurable therapeutic outcomes. Because the experiential aspects of occupation are not what we are used to as a source of satisfaction or because we are not sure if that is what is important or if that is what we can write down in our reports, we can be uneasy in these situations.

Of course, many of us are not working with people who have dementia or mental illness or are dying. Yet, I think that the importance of the experience of occupation applies to occupational therapy more broadly. The *experience* of occupation is thick with meaning; the experience of the therapy and occupation may, indeed, be the most potent source of satisfaction to the therapist and the client, in *all* therapy situations.

## THE THERAPIST AND THE SPLINT

One final story from my research with Virginia Dickie (Hasselkus & Dickie, 1994) illustrates the power of the experiential part of therapy for the therapist. The setting is an acute care hospital. The focus of the story is on a splint that the therapist devised to meet a patient's particular splinting needs as determined by the doctor. The product—the splint—is, of course, the doing part of the story. But listen to the voice of the therapist's occupational experience in this story as well—the therapist's own being, becoming, and belonging.

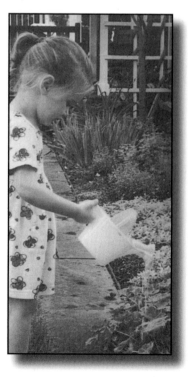

> We had gotten a call from a doctor and he's got this problem patient who he had done three surgeries on his forearm. He was very concerned about the patient moving [the arm] in the wrong way to jeopardize the surgery … he wanted him to be able to flex and extend his elbow to maintain that movement, but he didn't want him to pronate or supinate. So we were trying to come up with some sort of elbow-type deal that was also dynamic.
>
> I wound up fabricating—it was actually a two-piece, like a humeral cuff and like an ulnar cuff splint and made a hinge with it. Anyway, he [the patient] was able to flex and extend his elbow without any rotation at all.
>
> [*So far the emphasis in the story is on "doing" and the splint/product.*]
>
> And it was just a tedious splint. It took forever to make. It was just horrible; one of these nightmare splints that you've never made before.
>
> [*Now the experiential aspects of the situation have started to emerge as the therapist describes her state of mind, her way of "being" in the*

*situation—it was tedious, took forever, horrible, a nightmare, something she'd never done before.*]

Anyway, the next day the doctor had come in and wanted to know who made the splint. Of course we all panicked and pointed to me. And he just took me, shook my hand and just really praised me on what a good job it was and how effective it was.

[*More experiential expressions come through as the therapist describes the moment of panic felt by the therapists when the doctor asked who had made the splint; and then we can almost feel the relief she experienced when he went over to her, shook her hand, and told her "what a good job it was."*]

This was something that was really satisfying to me, being that I was able to really brainstorm, talk with the other therapists, come up with it, actually *make* it, and it actually *worked.* It looked good, too. That was a satisfying experience.

[*The therapist's own sense of well-being has surely been supported and enhanced by this experience, and it is likely that the splint-making experience has increased her self-confidence in this area of practice and her sense of her own ability to be creative and inventive has forged the beginnings of a close working relationship with one of the doctors, perhaps has even stimulated thoughts of specializing in splint-making. She is not the same therapist after this experience as she was before; the splint-making experience has moved her along in her development as an occupational therapist—has contributed to her "becoming" and to her "belonging" in the world of occupational therapy.*]

I propose that we are missing a lot by our tendency to focus so predominantly and sometimes almost exclusively on the doing aspects of our daily occupations—in our personal lives and in our work. I propose that it is in the experiencing of occupation that our own well-being and development and that of our clients are nurtured. The voice of occupation can be heard in both the everyday and the dramatic aspects of our lives—in the pincushions and thimbles, while watering the flowers and while making cookies, while inventing a new splint and while adapting a toothbrush. All of the days of our lives, occupation speaks.

As Eliot (1943) said, "Except for the point, the still point, there would be no dance." For me, there the dance is; and, after all, there *is* only the dance.

# REFERENCES

Eliot, T. S. (1943). *Four quartets.* New York, NY: Harcourt Brace Jovanovich.

Hasselkus, B. R., & Dickie, V. A. (1994). Doing occupational therapy: Dimensions of satisfaction and dissatisfaction. *American Journal of Occupational Therapy, 48,* 145-154.

Lydon, S. G. (1997). *The knitting sutra: Craft as a spiritual practice.* San Francisco, CA: Harper Collins.

# INDEX

abled gaze, 78
action. *See* performance
active living, 87–89, 90, 97
activity, related to occupation, 22, 23
acute medical crisis, as disability
   experience, 128, 129–130, 133–134
adversarial view of illness and disability,
   127–133, 136–138
adversity, creativity from, 177–178
affiliation cycles, 79
aging-in-place, 45
architecture, 43–44, 46
art therapy, 30–31, 172, 174–175, 176
aspect-blindness, 9–10
aspect-dawning, 8–9, 10
at-risk populations, 23, 32–33, 34
authentic selfhood, 25, 26–29, 172, 175
authentic understanding, 6, 7–8
autobiographical insideness, 47, 50, 51
average life theme, 134–135

balancing disability and ability, 125,
   128–129, 136, 137–138
balancing the unique and the shared,
   4–5, 6, 69–70, 103–106, 108–110,
   113–118, 119, 146
becoming, 24–25, 29–32, 67, 92, 93–96,
   150, 153, 187
being, 24–29, 150, 157–158, 186–187
belonging, 24–25, 32–34, 56, 67, 69, 71,
   73, 77, 106, 135, 153, 187
body movement, in space, 43–44
body-centered process, 49
boundaries, in organizational structures,
   33–34, 118
brainstorming, 169, 187
breach of reality, 77–78, 79
bridge, therapist as, 136–138, 175
Burns, George, 177–178

calculative thinking, 14
categories, in disability, 78, 79, 132–133
chaos, 50, 71, 170–171, 172, 176–178
children, and culture, 69–70, 178, 185
children, experience of place, 41, 42, 47,
   53–55
children, play experiences of, 111, 154,
   176
client-centered therapy, 29–30, 31,
   112–113, 149, 176
cognitive sets or biases, 169, 171
community, definitions of, 113
community spaces, 43–44, 45, 51, 54,
   55, 56
conformity, 5, 6, 70, 178–179
connection
   belonging, 24–25, 32–34, 56, 67, 69,
      71, 73, 77, 106, 135, 153, 187
   creativity, 70, 146, 166–168, 170, 171,
      172, 173–174, 175–176, 178–179
   culture, 3, 5, 67, 68–70, 103–106,
      113–117, 119
   disability, 11, 33–34, 115–116, 118,
      137–138
   duality of occupation for good or bad,
      109–113, 119
   institutional settings, 21–22, 25,
      33–34, 50–51, 109–111, 115–118,
      170
   meaning-giver, occupational therapist
      as, 21–22, 34
   narrative storytelling, 10–11, 12, 13,
      29, 113
   objectivism, 103–106, 113–116
   occupation, definitions of, 23, 25, 32
   occupational injustice, 23, 32–34
   overconnectedness, 107–108, 118,
      119
   personal and social meanings, 3, 4–5,
      6, 7, 26

shifting views on, 23, 105, 112–113
social support theory, 106–107
solitude, 108–110
spirituality, 106, 146, 147–148, 151,
    152–154, 155, 156–158
unfolding of therapist-client
    interaction, 11, 29–32
well-being, theories of, 86, 87–89, 90,
    91
context, in meaning-making, 3, 7, 9
continuity, 47, 56, 93, 109, 153–154
convergence, in rehabilitation process,
    134, 136
co-occupation, 112
creativity
    chaos, 170–171, 172, 176–178
    cognitive processes, 168–170, 171,
        173
    connection, 70, 146, 166–168, 170,
        171, 172, 173–174, 175–176,
        178–179
    constraints, 165, 166, 167, 168, 169,
        171, 172, 173, 178–179
    culture, 70, 72, 94, 171, 178
    definition of, 165
    disability, 176, 177–178
    in everyday life, 94, 165, 166, 170,
        171, 172–174, 175, 177–178, 179
    experience of occupation, 94, 187
    health and well-being, 172–178, 179
    space and place, 55, 166–167
    spirituality, 94, 151, 152, 158, 166,
        167, 172–173, 174
cultural competence, 66
culture
    connection, 3, 5, 67, 68–69, 103–106,
        113–117, 119
    creativity, 70, 72, 94, 171, 178
    cultivating difference in our lives,
        70–71
    cultivating the similar in our lives,
        67–70
    definitions of, 63, 65
    disability, 76–80, 125, 127–128
    experience of occupation, 185–186

health and well-being, 5, 7–8, 74–76,
    77, 78–79, 87–89, 116–117, 127,
    133–135
human development, 4, 5, 7, 79, 92,
    94–95, 116–117, 185
occupation, meaning of, 5, 22, 23, 66
routines, habits, and rituals, 66, 67,
    68, 85, 87
    definitions of, 71–72
    disability as occupational
        experience, 133–135, 136
    human development, 94, 96, 136
    liberation, 72–73, 155–156
    manageability, 74, 89–90
    occupation as disability experience,
        129–130, 132
    professional health care rituals,
        74–76
    space and place, 27, 41, 44, 45, 48,
        51
    spirituality, 94, 148, 152, 153,
        155–156
    symbolic meanings, 68, 72, 73–74,
        75, 76
as similarity and difference, 63–66,
    69–70
space and place, 27, 42–43, 44, 48,
    50, 69–70, 167
spirituality, 78, 94, 149, 153–154,
    155–156, 158

"dancing star," 170, 179
death and dying
    culture, 4, 5, 7–8, 67–69, 70, 105,
        114, 127, 185–186
    objectivism, 103–104, 105, 114
    as occupational experience, 6, 7, 135–
        136, 185–186
    personal and social meanings, 4, 5, 6,
        7–8, 9–10
    social support theory, 106–107
    space and place, 51–52
    spirituality, 147–148, 152–153, 156,
        157
    well-being, 85, 97, 106–107

decision making, 30, 31, 32, 33–34, 76, 78, 112–113, 115, 118, 168
deeper threads of difference, 64–65, 68
dehumanization, 50, 114, 132–133
delay of closure, 168
development
  becoming, 24–25, 29–32, 67, 92, 93–96, 150, 153, 187
  culture, 4, 5, 7, 79, 92, 94–95, 116–117, 185
  disability, 78–79, 126–127, 128, 131, 134, 138
  letting your life speak, 26–29, 93, 96
  lifespan context, 4–6, 10, 86, 91–96, 97, 147
  occupation, meaning of, 24–25
  as occupational experience, 185, 187
  personal and social meanings, 4–6, 7, 11, 45
  spirituality, 94, 146, 147, 155–156, 157
  transformative processes, 29, 92, 93–96, 148, 172, 177–178, 185
deviance, creativity as, 178–179
DeVries, Diane, 78
difference, cultivating, 70–71
directive approach to therapy, 29–30, 31
disability
  connection, 11, 33–34, 115–116, 118, 137–138
  creativity, 176, 177–178
  culture, 76–80, 125, 127–128
  faces of, 126–129, 137–138
  occupation as disability experience, 125, 129–133, 138
  as occupational experience, 125, 133–136, 138
  occupational injustice, 32, 33–34
  spirituality, 78, 156
disconnectedness
  culture, 103–106, 113–117, 119
  occupation as cause of, 109–110, 119
  occupational injustice, 32–34
  occupational therapy, 103–106, 113–116, 119
  organizational structure, 118

solitude, 108–110
spirituality, 146, 148
discontinuities, 170–171, 176
divergent thinking, 168, 169, 170
diversity, 66, 71, 112, 127
"doing,"
  connection, 109–111
  culture, 64, 65, 67, 71
  occupation, meaning of, 6–8, 24–25, 31–32, 46, 85, 109, 186–187
  spirituality, 150, 151–152
dual nature of occupational therapy, 114–116, 136–138
duality of occupation for good or bad, 109–110, 119
dynamic view of cultural change, 66

embracing properties, in homeyness, 49
environment. *See* space and place
ESM (experience sampling method), 13
ethnocentrism, 64, 65
ethnographic research, 11–12, 89–90, 104
experience of occupation, 3, 4–5, 7, 24, 94–96, 97, 185–187
experience sampling method (ESM), 13
expert, therapist as, 29–30, 31
expertise, development of, 5–6
expressive meaning, 14

family-centered care, 113
feng shui, 42–43
fractals, 171
frames, of life experiences, 5, 10, 11, 12, 67, 128, 156, 170
freeing, habits and routines as, 72–73
freeing of spirit, 151, 154–156, 157, 158
functional fixity, 169

genealogy, 52
geography of health, 55–56
globalization, 23
goals, 11, 30
  connection, 34, 112, 115–116, 118
  creativity, 165, 175
  culture, 7, 79, 116, 185

definition of, 27
disability, 78–79, 127, 138
versus letting your life speak, 26–27, 29
space and place, 34, 45, 118
spirituality, 146, 147
good life, concept of, 86, 88, 89, 90, 97
grounded theory, 11–12

habits, 44, 45, 71–73, 74, 96, 134, 135, 155–156
happiness, 21–22, 25, 27, 28, 87, 154, 174
health and well-being
    adversarial view of illness and disability, 127–133, 136–138
    connection
        duality of occupation for good or bad, 109–113, 119
        ideology of independence, 116–117
        institutional settings, 33–34, 51, 115–118
        objectivism, 103–106, 113–116
        occupational injustice, 23, 32–34
        overconnectedness, 107–108, 118, 119
        shared stories, 11, 113
        social support theory, 106–107
        solitude, 108–110
        therapeutic relationship, 4, 5–6, 7–8, 11, 22, 90–91, 103–105, 111–116, 119
    creativity, 172–178, 179
    culture, 5, 7–8, 74–76, 77, 78–79, 87–89, 116–117, 127, 133–135
    ill-being, 22, 91
    lifespan human development, 92, 93
    occupation, meaning of, 23, 24, 85, 96–97, 113, 187
    space and place, 27, 42–43, 46, 55–56, 86, 87–88, 89, 91, 117–118
    spirituality, 87, 106, 146–148, 152, 154, 155, 157
    theories of well-being, 86–91, 97
health promoting responses, 134, 136, 175

heirlooms, 153–154
Hmong culture, 75–76
holistic health view, 126–127, 128, 129, 136–138
home, 43, 44–45, 46–51, 52, 53, 55–56, 118, 166–167
home designs or modifications, 44
homelessness, 32, 33, 118
homesickness, 43
homeyness, 41, 49–50, 51, 53
humanness, loss of, 50, 114, 132–133

identity, 85, 103
    creativity, 176, 178
    culture, 64, 65, 95
    definition of, 26
    disability, 127, 132–133, 135
    human development, 93, 95
    space and place, 46, 47, 50, 56
    spirituality, 147
ill health, creativity from, 172, 176–178
ill-being, 22, 91
independence, as cultural value, 5, 23, 66, 73, 116–117
inner being, 26–27, 28, 29, 95, 145–146, 152
inside room, spirituality as, 145–146, 151, 152, 157
institutional settings, 186–187
    connection, 21–22, 25, 33–34, 50–51, 109–111, 115–118, 170
    creativity, 21–22, 24–25, 30–31, 168, 169, 170, 175
    health and well-being, 21–22, 24–25, 27, 55–56, 74–76
    two-body practice in occupational therapy, 115–116, 137
integrative thinking, 14
interactive reasoning, 112
interpretive (qualitative) research, 11–12, 13
intrinsicality, 150
isolation. *See* disconnectedness; solitude

Japanese Kawa (river) model, 92, 116, 117, 119

kitchen, as place, 44, 47–48
"knowing" meaning, 10–13
knowing one's self, 25–26, 27, 28
knowledge in integrative thinking, 14
knowledge units of everyday experiences, 10

lateral thinking, 168–169, 170
leisure, 23–24, 25, 148
letting your life speak, 26–29, 93, 96
life transitions therapy, 92–93
lifespan human development, 4–6, 10, 86, 91–96, 97, 147
lived experience over time and space (space-time depth), 46, 48, 50, 52, 114–116
logico-scientific mode of thought, 14

manageability, 74, 89–90, 91
marked categories, 132–133
meaningfulness, 13, 22, 25, 28, 42, 89, 90, 91
meaning-givers, 21–22, 34
meaninglessness, 4
medical crisis, as disability experience, 129–130
medical geography, 55–56
medical models of illness and disability, 127–133, 136–138, 156
meditative thinking, 14
memories of experience, 41–42, 45, 47, 51, 54–55
metaphoric understanding, 170
mindfulness and mindlessness, 9–10
minimal well-being, 91
"mirror phenomenon," in understanding disability, 77–78
moirés, 11
Montaigne, Michel de, 84, 85, 97, 129

narratives/storying of life experiences
   connection, 10–11, 12, 13, 29, 113
   disability, 11, 134–135, 178
   how we "know" meaning, 10–12, 13, 14
   space and place, 45, 47, 52
   spirituality, 151, 152, 153–154, 156–157

"normal" part of life, disability as, 126–127, 128, 129
nuances, sensitivity to, 170

objectified research, 12–13
objectivism, 103–106, 113–116
occupation, related to activity, 22, 23
occupational apartheid, 23
occupational categories, 9, 23–24
occupational deprivation, 23
occupational forms, 12–13, 109–113
occupational injustice, 23, 32–34
occupational performance, 6–8, 12, 13, 43, 46, 148, 149, 155
occupational rights, 23
occupational spin-off, 90
occupationally experienced, disability as, 133–136
offices, as place, 47, 53, 166–167
open door policy, 14
ordinary language, 12
organizational creativity, 168
Osgood's Meaning Differential, 12
"otherness" concept, 63, 64, 70–71, 73, 76
overconnectedness, 107–108, 118, 119

paradox of disability, 79–80, 125
paradox of rehabilitation, 78–79, 80, 138
partner, therapist as, 29–30, 31
performance, 6–8, 12, 13, 43, 46, 148, 149, 155
personal meanings
   aspects of seeing, 8–10
   culture, 5, 22, 23, 66, 73, 116
   dynamic process of construction, 3, 5, 10
   frames, of life experiences, 5, 10, 11, 12, 67, 128, 156, 170
   novice to expert, 5–6
   place memories, 41–42, 45
   and social meanings, continuum of, 4–5, 6
   spirituality, 146, 147, 148, 153–154
   *See also* home; narratives/storying of life experiences

person-centered process, 48–49
phenomenological occupation and the person, 95–96
phenomenological research, 11–12
phenomenological views of the body, 114–116, 137
physical illness, creativity from, 172, 176–178
place. See space and place
place integration, 7, 45, 51
place memories, 41–42, 45
placelessness, 45–46, 51, 55–56
populations, at-risk, 23, 32–33, 34
positive human health, 86–87, 88, 90, 97
power, in organizational structures, 33–34, 118
practical knowledge, 5–6
presencing, 147–148
problem solving, 168–169
purpose in life, 13, 22, 23, 24, 26, 86–87, 91, 106, 145, 147, 156, 185

reality, breach in, 77–78, 79
real-world knowledge, 10, 11
rebellion, creativity as, 172, 178
rehabilitation
    balancing disability and ability, 137–138
    convergence process, 134, 136
    culture, 77, 78–79, 80, 116–117, 127–128
    loss of humanness, 132–133
    spirituality, 148, 150
relational space, 56
relational view of creativity, 167–168
relationships. See connection
relative well-being, 91, 110–111
release of spirit, 151, 154–156, 157, 158
research approaches on meaning and occupation, 11–13
rich points, culture revealed in, 63–64, 65, 67
rituals
    culture, related to, 67, 68, 69, 71, 72, 135
    human development, 94, 96

professional health care, 74–76
    space and place, 41
    spirituality, 94, 148, 155
    symbolic meanings, 68, 72, 73–74, 75, 76
river (Kawa) model, 92, 116, 117, 119
river delta metaphor, 21
room metaphor for spirituality, 145–146, 151, 152, 157
room of one's own, 52–53, 55, 118, 167
routines, 85, 87
    culture, related to, 66, 67, 71–73, 135
    disability as occupational experience, 133–135, 136
    human development, 96, 136
    manageability, 74, 89–90
    mindfulness, 9
    occupation as disability experience, 129–130, 132
    space and place, 27, 41, 45, 48, 51
    spirituality, 152, 153, 155–156

Sarton, May, 108, 109, 110
scientific method, 4, 105, 106, 149
search for meaning in life, 3, 5, 46, 92, 118, 146, 153
seeing, aspects of, 8–10, 56, 78
self, 85, 103, 106
    creativity, 168–170, 171, 172, 173, 175, 178, 179
    culture, 63–65, 67, 70–71
    definition of, 25, 26
    home, 47, 48–49, 50, 51
    knowing one's self, 25–26, 27, 28
    selfing, 26, 31–32, 93
    solitude, 108–110
    spirituality, 146, 147–148, 151, 153
    See also being; development; identity; personal meanings
self-care, 23–24, 25, 72, 109, 116–117
sense of coherence, 89–90
sensitive dependence on initial conditions, 171
situated meaning, 3, 7
situational diagnosis, 33–34, 118
social networks, 106–107, 154, 167

social relationships. *See* connection; culture
social support theory, 106–107
social-centered process, 48, 49
solitude, 108–110
space and place
    creativity, 55, 166–167
    culture, 27, 42–43, 44, 48, 50, 69–70, 167
    definitions of, 41–42
    health and well-being, 27, 42–43, 46, 55–56, 86, 87–88, 89, 91, 117–118
    home, 43, 44–45, 46–51, 52, 53, 55–56, 118, 166–167
    meanings, 7, 32, 33–34, 41–42, 45, 46–53
    occupational therapy, 7, 43–45, 46, 49, 56
    placelessness, 45–46, 51, 55–56
    room of one's own, 52–53, 55, 118, 167
    special places, 51–55
    spirituality, 145–146, 151, 152, 153, 157–158
space within, spirituality as, 157–158
space-time depth, 46, 48, 50, 52
spirit, release of, 151, 154–156, 157, 158
spiritual distress, 146, 147, 157
spirituality
    connection, 106, 146, 147–148, 151, 152–154, 155, 156–158
    creativity, 94, 151, 152, 158, 166, 167, 172–173, 174
    culture, 78, 94, 149, 153–154, 155–156, 158
    disability, 78, 156
    everyday occupation, 149, 150–154, 158
    health and well-being, 87, 106, 146–148, 152, 154, 155, 157
    human development, 94, 146, 147, 155–156, 157
    inside room metaphor for, 145–146, 151, 152, 157
    occupational therapy, 148–150, 151, 154–157, 158
    as space within, 157–158

stories. *See* narratives/storying of life experiences
surveillance zones, 56
swing memory, 41, 42, 54
symbolic meanings
    culture, related to, 63, 66, 67
    rituals, 68, 72, 73–74, 75, 76
    space and place, 45, 47, 49, 52–53, 56
    spirituality, 94, 153–154

technology, 79, 105–106, 108, 114, 119, 171
thematic meaning, 14
theoretical knowledge, 5–6
therapeutic landscapes, 42
therapeutic occupation, 12
therapeutic relationship as connectedness, 111–113
therapist-client interaction, unfolding of, 11, 29–32
threads of difference, 64–65, 68
total institutions, 50–51
transactionalism, 43, 56, 157
transformative processes, 29, 92, 93–96, 148, 172, 177–178, 185
transitional therapy, 92–93
two-body practice in occupational therapy, 114–116, 136–138

visitation event, 67–68, 69, 70
visual field of home, 56

webs of significance, 63, 64, 68–69
well-being. *See* health and well-being
well-elderly study, 90–91
Woolf, Virginia, 52–53
work, as occupation, 23–24, 25, 148
work spaces, 47, 53, 166–167

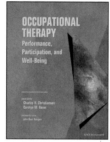
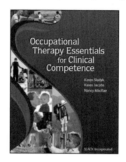

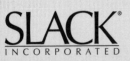